A colour atlas of

Physical Signs in General Medicine

M. ZATOUROFF
M.R.C.P. Lond.

WOLFE MEDICAL PUBLICATIONS LTD

Copyright © M Zatouroff, 1976
Published by Wolfe Medical Publications Ltd, 1976
Printed by Grafos, Arte Sobre Papel, Barcelona, Spain
9th impression 1989
ISBN 0 7234 0185 3 Cased edition
ISBN 0 7234 0864 5 Limp edition

General Editor, Wolfe Medical Books
G Barry Carruthers MD(Lond)

This book is one of the titles in the series of
Wolfe Medical Atlases, a series which brings together
probably the world's largest systematic published
collection of diagnostic colour photographs.

For a full list of Atlases in the series, plus
forthcoming titles and details of our surgical, dental
and veterinary Atlases, please write to
Wolfe Medical Publications Ltd, Brook House,
2-16 Torrington Place, London WC1E 7LT.

Contents

To Diana, Anna, Justin and Catherine
without whose forbearance this book
would never have been finished

Introduction

General medicine overlaps into many different specialities: the aim of this book is to cover ground which is relevant and important to all specialities, though aspects which are essentially general surgery have been omitted. The photographs show the appearance of a physical sign at the bedside and cover the minimal as well as the gross entity, so that the full spectrum can be appreciated. In some sections several pictures of the same condition are provided, so that the characteristic 'face' of the disease can be recognised.

The clinical undergraduate will be able to study a wide selection of short cases and a number of very common conditions are included. The postgraduate requires a different approach: some of the photographs suggest an 'approach to seeing' and a train of logical thought and correlation rather than spot diagnosis. For both the undergraduate and the postgraduate the illustrations provide useful comparisons with the colour slides which are used more and more in examinations.

A section on folk medicine and customs amongst different races is also included. This serves to bring to the student's attention the diagnostic significance of certain burns, scars and stains.

The format of the book follows the head-to-foot sequence of physical examination. This means that some pictures which relate to a certain condition may be spread throughout the book. The captions begin with the diagnosis, describe the picture in order to heighten attention and bring out detail, and the student can then adopt this approach when he sees an abnormality which he does not recognise. Where it seemed relevant, causes, differential diagnoses and additional points to look for have been mentioned.

The photographs were taken either at the bedside, or in the consulting room, using Kodachrome 11 film, and occasionally High Speed Ektachrome. The cameras were a Pentax and a Leicaflex with 60mm macro and 135mm lenses with close-up attachments. Electronic flash was used for most pictures, although the African photographs were taken in available light at an aperture of $f1.8$ and so have a very shallow depth of field. The patients, from West African to Arabian, Mediterranean and Anglo Saxon, represent a multi-racial collection, typical of general medicine.

The Approach to Photographs and Slides

Many examinations now use photographs and colour slides in order to test the knowledge of the student. Some practical approach is necessary since intuitive guessing is often wrong.

When you look at a photograph for the first time, always reconsider the first thing that comes to your mind and test it against logical deduction: if it appears wrong do not discard it totally, often the first thought *is* right! If you cannot identify the signs, either in a picture or in life, observe carefully and describe logically what you see. As you do this the story unfolds and when you reach the end you may realise that you have described the diagnosis.

The approach varies with experience. The undergraduate is happy with the diagnosis of the physical sign: *'clubbing'* for instance. The postgraduate should go further: if cyanosis is present, then *'clubbing in cyanotic congenital heart disease'*; if the fingers are heavily stained with nicotine, then *'clubbing in carcinoma of the bronchus'.* He sees another sign and relates the two together.

The first step is to describe accurately in simple words what is seen. Care is necessary to avoid using powerful, diagnostically emotive words in the description since it is then difficult to change your mind – for instance if a rash is described as butterfly it is extremely unlikely that anything other than the diagnosis of lupus erythematosus will finally emerge. The second point is that whilst describing what you see often the description will suddenly mean something and the diagnosis will come from the depths of your mind. Thirdly, once the diagnosis is established it is important not to describe what you do not see, but which does occur in the condition, in the mistaken belief that such display of knowledge will impress the examiner. It is useless to point out an enophthalmos in a case of Horner's syndrome (**267**) when it does not exist. Similarly it is difficult to see a difference in sweating or a change in temperature on an ordinary colour photograph.

When looking at a rash it should be described in simple terms, macular, papular, vesicular, or pustular and its distribution confirmed by thoughtful search. It is *not* localised if there are spots in another portion of the anatomy but *maximal* at that site (**740**).

Finally if there are two physical signs present they should be taken *separately,* the causes of each sign run over mentally, and where the causes coincide will be a logical suggestion for the diagnosis. This will reassure the examiner that the candidate thinks clearly, e.g.

(1) **266**: Horner's syndrome and trophic fingers. Horner's syndrome is due to a lesion of the cervical sympathetic chain anywhere in its course. If another sign suggests the level that will pinpoint the diagnosis, then:
   (1) could be – burns = syringo myelia
   (2) Raynaud's phenomenon = treated by sympathectomy
   (3) emboli = cervical rib
Only the first two relate to the Horner's syndrome (*syn.* Bernard-Horner syndrome) and are possible diagnoses.

(2) **277**: Hyperextension of the hip, which could be due to laxity, hypermobility or hypertonicity. The cause may be:
   (1) genetic – pseudoxanthoma elasticum and Ehlers Danlos syndrome
   (2) occupational – in the ballet dancer or acrobat
   (3) environmental in the Arab accustomed to sit cross-legged
   (4) neurological due to hypotonicity
   (5) anatomical due to joint destruction
But in addition bilateral ptosis is present – congenital, myopathic, myasthenic or tabetic in origin.

Diagnosis: probably tabes dorsalis.

The most important things are to look, describe and think. It is no good looking and expecting to find the diagnosis written on the patient's body, the diagnosis is there, all you have to do is to describe what you see.

(Johann Friedrich Horner, 1831–1886, described 1869; Claude Bernard, 1813–1878, described 1862; Edvard Ehlers, 1863–1937, described 1901; Henri Alexander Danlos, 1844–1912, described 1908.)

The Head

THE FACE

Observation of the facies, the expression, may give information about the patient's state of mind and physical health: mood or haemoglobin, health or disease, malnutrition or endocrine state. Clues are there to the system that is at fault.

1 *Health* Alert, bright-eyed, no pallor and normal skin turgor.

2 *Disease (carcinoma of the pancreas)* Apathetic and drowsy: loss of subcutaneous fat, sunken eyes and cheeks with loss of skin turgor secondary to dehydration. The picture of terminal illness.

3 *Pallor* This is not synonymous with anaemia since a pale skin may be due to depigmentation or vasoconstriction, apart from a fall in the haemoglobin concentration. Pallor of the skin must be confirmed by looking at the mucous membranes. Note: the colour of the skin; a slight malar flush with dilated superficial veins; a left sided corneal arcus; obesity – the roundness of the face which is not due to steroid therapy, but could be; the fact that the hair has been dyed (this is irrelevant but one should learn to observe everything).
    In fact this woman's haemoglobin was 14g% and this underlines the fallacy of using pallor as an index of anaemia. (See **4**).

4 *Pallor of the conjunctivae* Note the difference in colour between the examiner's nailbed and the conjunctival mucous membrane – one can be misled since this woman's haemoglobin was 14g%. Confirmation should be sought by examination of other mucous membranes and estimation of their degree of pallor.

1

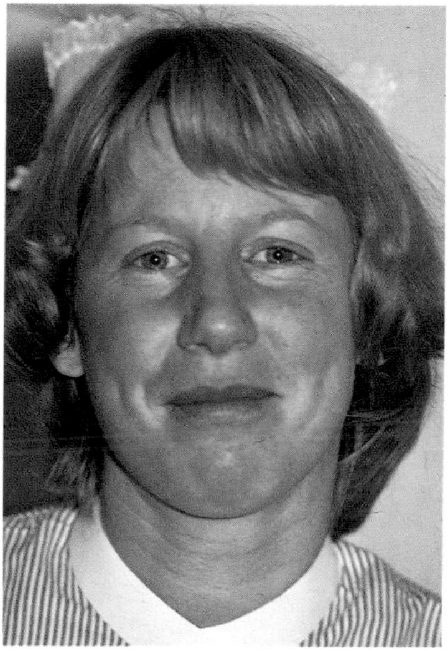

2

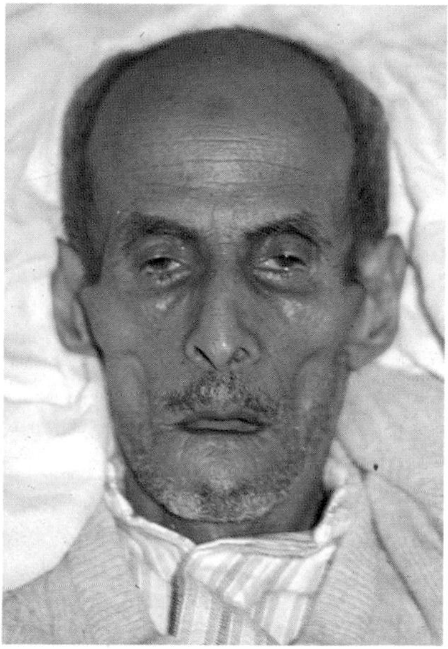

3

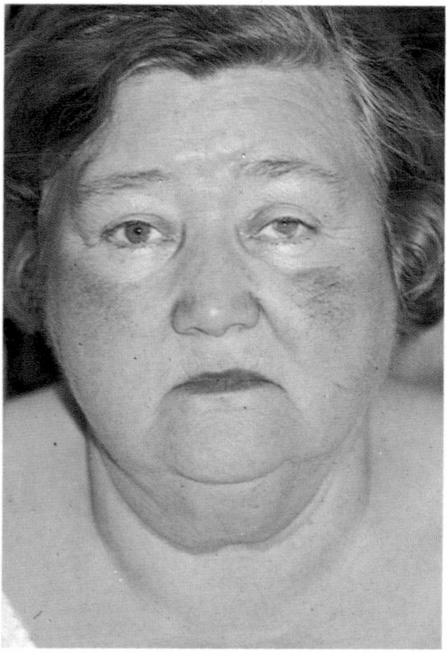

4

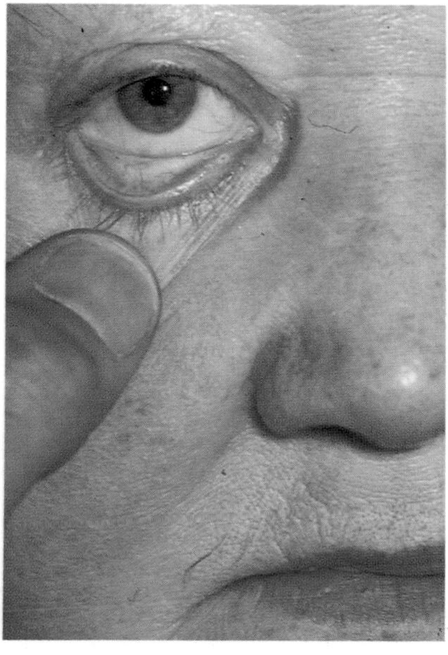

5 *Pallor (pernicious anaemia)* A woman of middle age. The lips and face are pale, the hair white, the eyes blue. Note the pallor of the lower lid margin, the tattoo on the left shoulder. This woman presents the classic clinical picture of the facies of pernicious anaemia.

6 *Pallor (pernicious anaemia)* Facial pallor, blue eyes, grey hair. Bilateral corneal arcus.

7 *Anaemia* This thin, pale woman with a scarred abdomen had a gastrectomy which produced her iron deficiency anaemia. Note the wasting, the abdominal scar and dilated veins which in her case are not significant. Dilated veins should always be observed since they may indicate a venous block in the deep circulation.

8 *Megaloblastic anaemia* Megaloblastic anaemia in the elderly, slight pallor, tinge of jaundice in the eye, atrophy of the tongue and healed angular stomatitis.

5

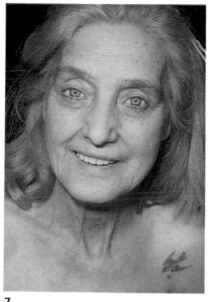

6

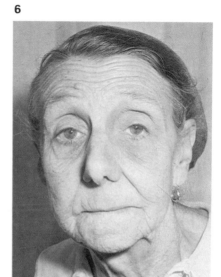

7

8

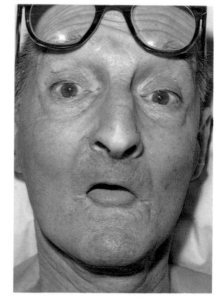

9 *Pallor (rectal bleeding)* Pale lips and face. This man looks ill and apathetic. Haemoglobin 6g%.

Diagnosis: carcinoma of the rectum; long standing diarrhoea secondary to ulcerative colitis. Compare his facies and alertness with the preceding plate where the haemoglobin was 5g% and with the pre and post transfusion appearance of the mucous membrane on the inside of the lower lip (**11** & **12**).

10 *Pallor of the conjunctivae in severe anaemia* The colour of the mucous membrane and the conjunctival sac is an index of the degree of anaemia but it may be reassuringly red in severe anaemia and should be compared with the inside of the lower lip.

11 *Pallor of the mucous membrane of the lower lip* Same patient as **10**, confirming the conjunctival impression of severe anaemia. Note the mild pyorrhoea, gum recession and nicotine staining of the teeth. This is a particularly reliable site to check for pallor and estimate the haemoglobin by contrast with the examiner's nailbed.

12 *Normal mucosa of the lower lip* The same patient, following transfusion of five pints of packed red cells.

9

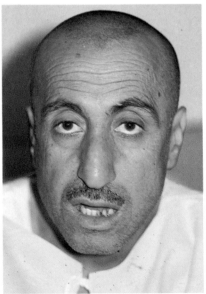

10

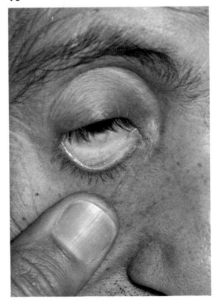

11

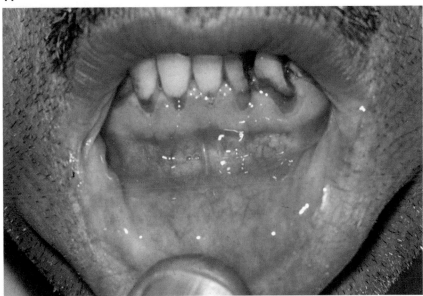

12

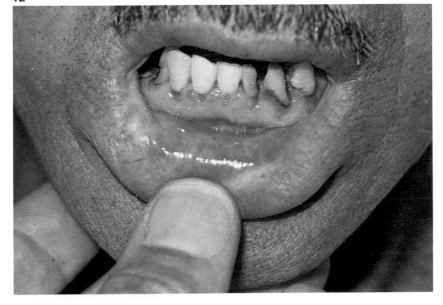

13

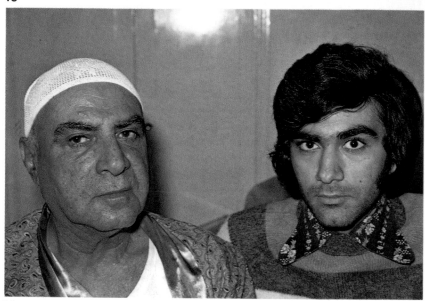

14

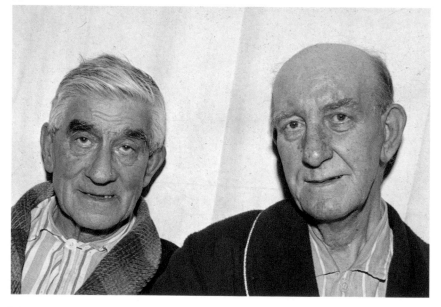

13 & 14 *Facial plethora (polycythaemia rubra vera)* On the left the man has a red face compared with the normal on the right. This facial plethora may be within normal limits or may be secondary to an increase in the number of red cells.

15 *Facial plethora* Healthy open air worker. Secondary facial plethora, normal haemoglobin.

16 *The anaemic Negro* In the Negro anaemia may present as a greyness of a black skin and the pallor is difficult to see. Haemoglobins of 5g% can be missed in active farmers with hookworm, whose anaemia has come on slowly and whose symptoms are minimal. One must be familiar with the nuances of colour change.
  Note the evidence of recent wasting in the folding of the skin.

15

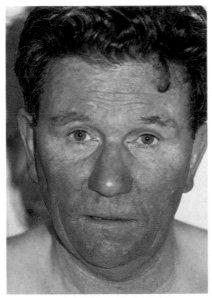

16

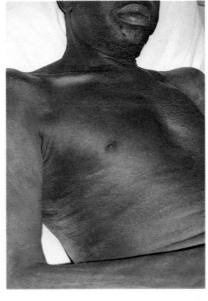

17 *A pale normal Negro* A Negro whose pigmentation is not dense and therefore looks pale compared with the previous picture. His conjunctivae are pink.

18 & 19 *A dark, anaemic Negro* A Negro with dark pigmentation who has pallor of the conjunctivae and a haemoglobin of 5g%. Compare this with his lower lip, where there is obvious yellow pallor of the inside of the lower lip. This is a markedly anaemic Negro.

20 *Pallor of the nailbeds contrasted with the normal* Haemoglobin: 6g%. Examination of the hands should include comparison with your own hand.

17

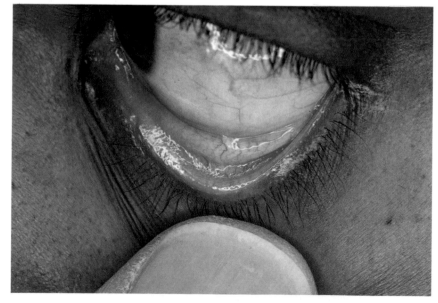

18

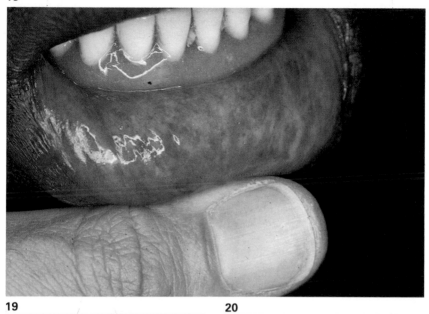

19

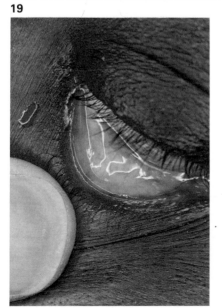

20

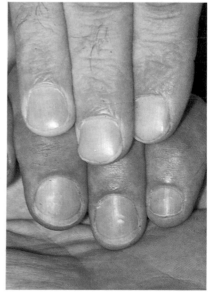

21 & 22 *Koilonychia (spoon shaped)* If you see pallor, look at the hands and nails. Koilonychia is associated with iron deficiency anaemia and hepatic disease. Classically, koilonychia is described as being able to take a drop of water in the depression of the nailbed.

23 *Malnutrition (child)* Complete picture of early protein/calorie malnutrition. General misery, wasting, oedema, pallor of the skin, fineness and depigmentation of the hair, puffiness of the face, and a protuberant belly.

21

22

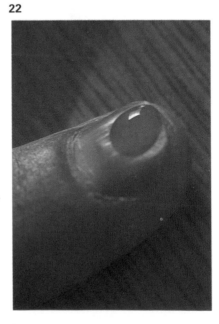

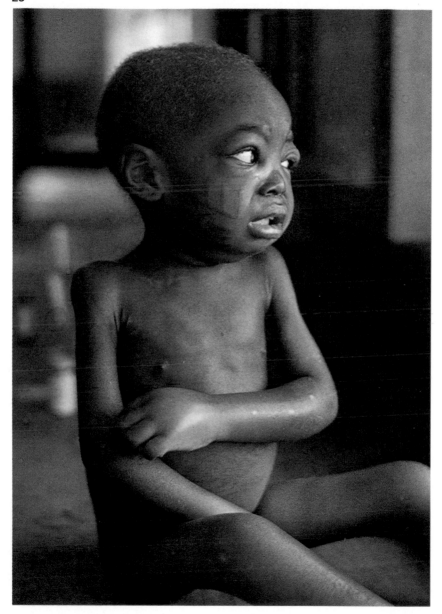

24 *Malnutrition (adult), famine starvation* Depigmentation of the hair, pale skin. The scars are of tribal cosmetic significance. Yoruba, western region Nigeria.

25 *Kwashiorkor (protein/calorie malnutrition)* Note the oedema, scaliness, depigmentation. (See **26**).

26 *Kwashiorkor* As the skin peels an ooze of fluid appears and leads to further loss of protein.

27 *Malnutrition* The tongue is smooth and shiny, has lost its normal furred papillae and splitting of the corners of the mouth is noted. There is also a characteristic scaling of the skin and depigmentation over the nose in a patient with severe malnutrition.

28 *Malnutrition* A Nigerian with malabsorption following gastrectomy, pallor, wasting and skin changes of protein deficiency: cracking of the skin and pigmentation.

24

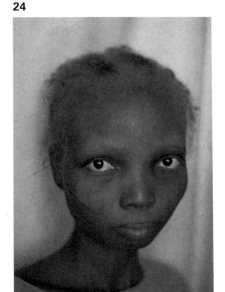

25

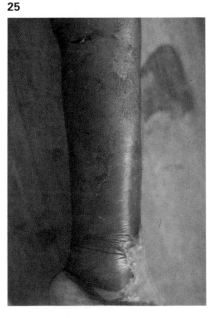

26

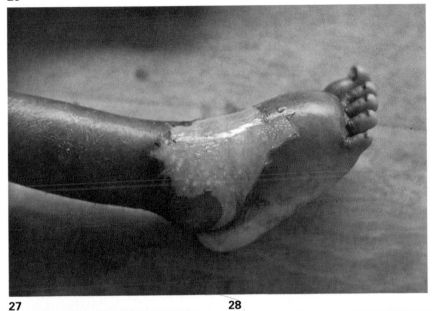

27

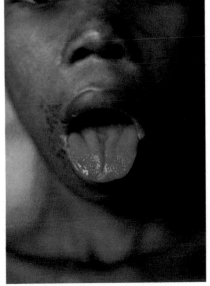

28

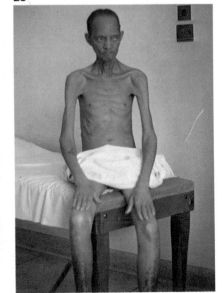

29 *Anaemia, telangiectasia of the tongue* This patient presented with anaemia. Apart from slight pallor there were no obvious physical signs, there are healed scars at the corners of the mouth and two small telangiectases can be seen on the left cheek. When the tongue was examined the telangiectases were easily seen.

30 & 31 *Congenital telangiectasia* The telangiectases may be seen on the face, around the angle of the jaw and are well seen on the ear.

32 *Telangiectasia* This man, who has telangiectasia seen round the borders of the lips, presented initially with haematemesis and over the course of years had a gastrectomy followed by the malabsorption complications of gastrectomy and developed tuberculosis. It was only when he shaved off his exuberant moustache that the telangiectasia was noted.

29

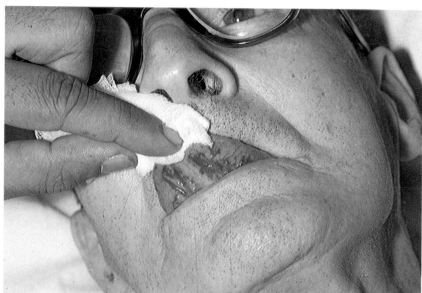

30

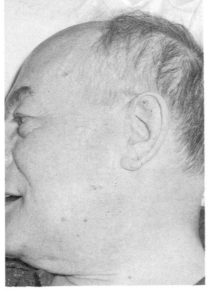

31

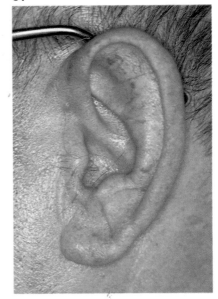

32

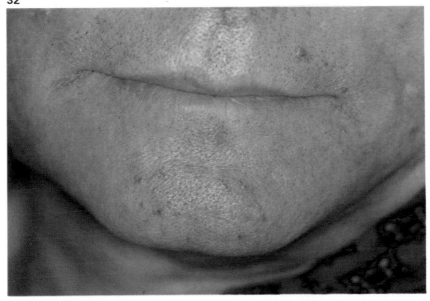

33 *Telangiectasia* On the inside of the lower lip telangiectases may be more obvious. Dilated capillaries are well seen and the capillary loop in the middle is obvious.

34 *Sickle cell anaemia* Note the pallor, the prominent forehead due to expansion of the bones of the skull. A tint of jaundice can be seen in the conjunctivae. This appearance may be seen in Mediterranean anaemia and other haemoglobinopathies where there is a hypertrophy of the bone marrow. The scars on the cheeks are Yoruba tribal markings in the African.

35 *Sickle cell anaemia* Dactylitis in a small child with bone infarction producing an acute, tender swelling of the finger. Differential diagnosis between sepsis, acute or chronic (tuberculosis), syphilis, sickle cell disease, sarcoidosis.

36 *The malar flush* The redness of the cheeks may be seen in health. There is a clinical association between this physical sign and mitral stenosis but it also may be seen in polycythaemia, in steroid therapy, and in outdoor workers.

37 *Frank jaundice of the eyes* Dehydration, emaciation, carcinoma of pancreas. Bilirubin 8mg%.

33

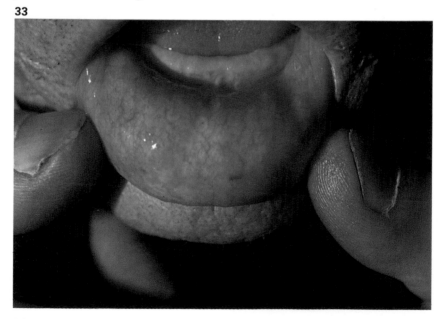

34

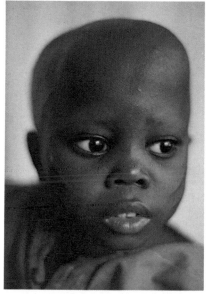

35

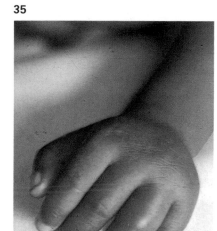

36

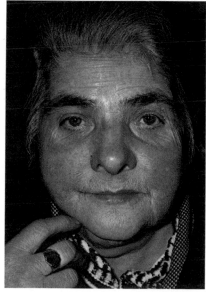

37

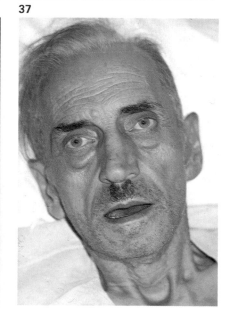

38 *A tinge of jaundice* Bilirubin 2mg%. The tinge compared with the normal lady on the right. Best seen in the conjunctivae.

39 *Jaundice* The shininess of the nail due to the polishing effect of using the fingers to scratch the back which itched. Patient was a 42-year-old man with a stone in a common bile duct.

Note the polished nail *tip* is caused by scratching the skin. Cosmetic polishing makes the whole nail shine. Pruritus may be due to: (1) parasitic infestations: scabies, pediculosis; (2) eczema; (3) liver disease (even preceding jaundice); (4) drug reactions; (5) malignant disease (lymphoma, leukaemia, carcinoma); (6) metabolic disease (diabetes mellitus, uraemia); (7) old age.

40 *Excoriations of the back secondary to scratching (primary biliary cirrhosis)* The excoriations all occur in those parts of the back within reach. This physical sign may be seen before the development of other physical signs of liver disease, and precede the jaundice.

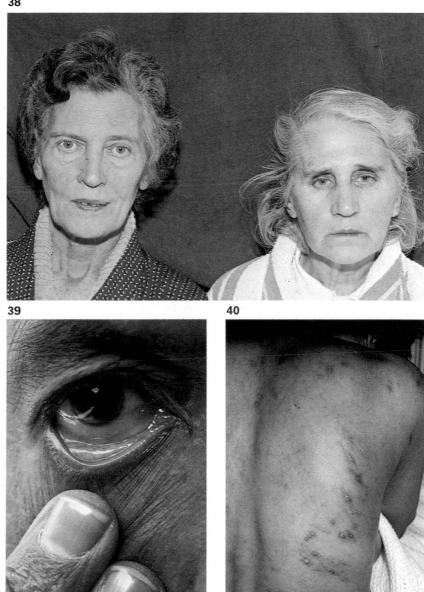

38

39

40

41 *Spider naevus on the nose* Note the central vessel and the peripheral erythema. Pressure on the central vessel produced blanching and release demonstrated the capillary branches from the central arteriole. This condition of spider naevi is usually seen above the nipples and may occur physiologically and pathologically: (1) in pregnancy; (2) in normal women, increasing at the time of period; (3) in high output states; (4) in liver disease.

This young girl developed a spider naevus during the first month of her pregnancy and it increased in size to term and began to diminish in size within hours of delivery of her baby.

42 *Spider naevus* A central feeding vessel can be seen, surrounded by a small zone of erythema. This will blanch on pressure and will reappear from the centre when the pressure is released.

43 *Campbell de Morgan spots* These are frequently seen, increasing in middle age and in the elderly. Flat, slightly raised spots which do not blanch on pressure and have no central arteriole and must not be confused with spider naevi. They are of no significance.

44 *Palmar erythema* This is an increase in the erythema of the palms, usually localised on the thenar and hypothenar eminences. It occurs in the healthy adult, frequently in pregnancy, and in association with liver disease, rheumatoid arthritis and thyrotoxicosis. In this picture one can also see an early Dupuytren's contracture developing in the palm. The palms are warm and may even have a burning quality. Areas of erythema are also seen at the base of the fingers. The erythema blanches on pressure. This patient suffered from cirrhosis of the liver and drank one and a half bottles of whisky daily. *(Guillaume Dupuytren, 1777–1835, described 1831.)*

41

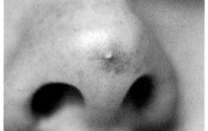

42

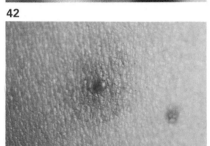

43

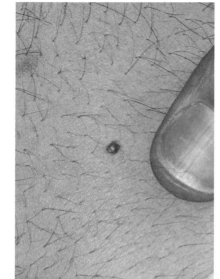

44

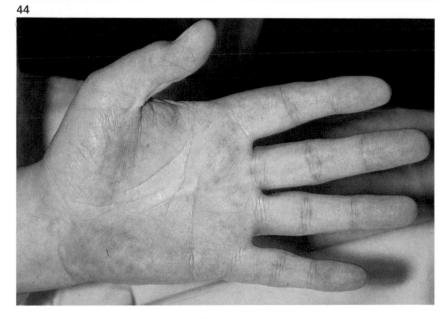

45 *White nails* Although described in cirrhosis it is not diagnostic and is seen in a variety of conditions. Best seen here in the third finger (normal below). The whiteness of the nail due to opacification of the nailbed diminishes as the tip is reached and a pink rim can be seen in the right hand finger (ring finger). Note that the lunula cannot be seen compared with the normal.

45

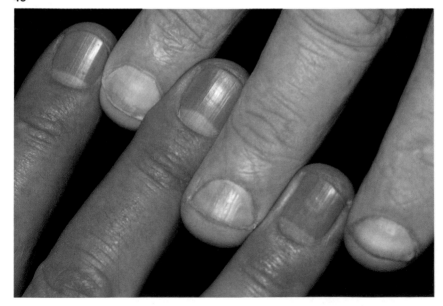

Colour changes in the skin

Secondary to change in haemoglobin
pallor
   changes in Hb concentration or
   changes in Hb supply to skin (vasoconstriction)
plethora
cyanosis
   peripheral – vasoconstriction, stagnation
   central – shunts, anoxia, sulph and methaemoglobinaemia
carbon dioxide poisoning

Hypopigmentation
albino
vitiligo
irradiation

Hyperpigmentation
sunlight
racial
von Recklinghausen's disease
melanosis
haemochromatosis
thyrotoxicosis
ACTH administration
hypoadrenocorticalism (Addison's disease)

Other pigments deposited in the skin
bilirubin
carotene
drugs: mepacrine
metals: lead, mercury, gold
arsenic

Miscellaneous
malnutrition
chloasma of pregnancy

Surface applications
cosmetics and perfumes
silver nitrate – silver deposited
pot. permanganate – reacts with keratin, difficult to remove

46–49 *Haemochromatosis* A man of middle age who had mild diabetes, loss of hair on the chest and in the axilla, and hepato-splenomegaly. There is no forearm hair, the skin is thin, and there are no creases of the arm. Almost a pigmented hypopituitary state! The slate grey colouration of the skin is secondary to the melanin and haemosiderin deposition and thinning of the epidermis. The pigment may have brown tinge and patches may be seen in the oral mucosa.

Figure **48** shows the slate grey skin of haemochromatosis compared with normal skin, and **49** is a close-up of the skin of the chest showing very fine, downy hair.

50 *Haemochromatosis* Chondrocalcinosis in haemochromatosis, in the cartilage overlying the metacarpo-phalangeal joints of the fingers. No evidence of hyperparathyroidism, gout or pseudo gout, osteo arthritis, Wilson's disease, all of which may be associated with calcification in cartilage.

46

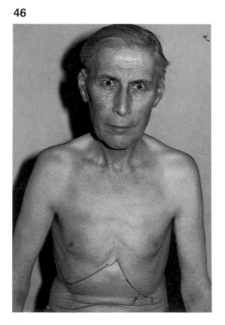

47

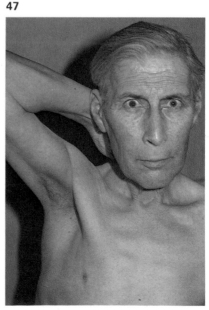

48

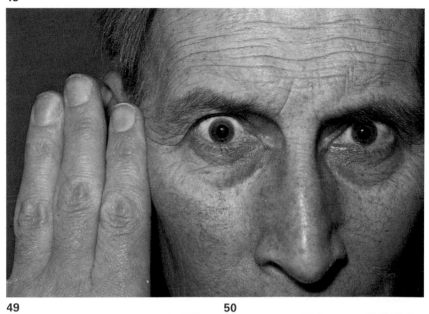

49

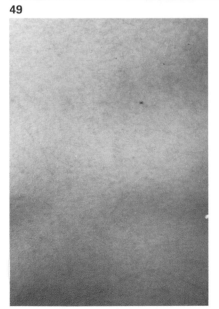

50

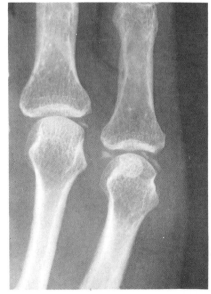

51 *Melanosis in melanomatosis* Secondary melanoma of the orbit. True pigmentation of a slate colour, both of the site of the secondary tumour and strikingly of the skin. This slate grey pigmentation is a darker colour than the pigmentation of haemochromatosis.

52 *Melanosis (patient and control)* Widespread secondary melanoma with liberated pigment staining the skin.

53 *Melanoma in abdominal scar* Note the grey pigment showing through in the upper and lower thirds of the wound. This patient presented with a gland under the left arm and gave a story of removal of a thumb nail several years earlier which may have been the primary. The gland was removed, block dissection of the axilla carried out and one year later he presented with intestinal obstruction and at operation had secondaries throughout the small bowel, some of them obstructing and about to perforate.

54 *Caroteneaemia* Yellow pigmentation due to carotene. This is caused by (1) excess carotene intake – overeating mangoes, carrots (4kg a day!), pawpaw, oranges; (2) myxoedema – high levels of carotene due to a defect of enzymatic conversion to vitamin A; (3) an association with hyperbetalipoproteinaemia.

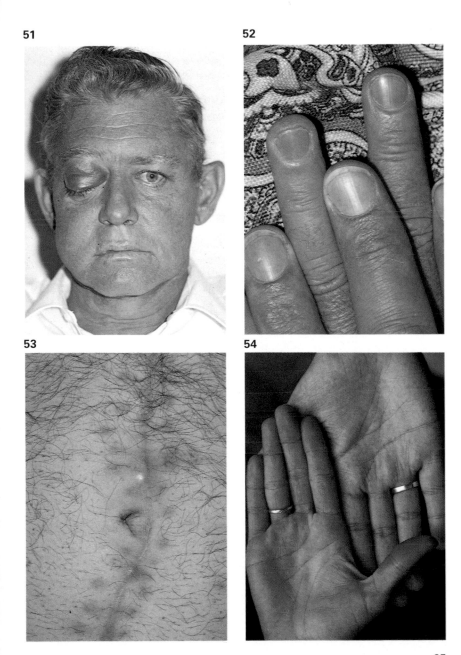

55–58 *Vitiligo* Vitiligo of the face with depigmentation around the eyes and mouth in a healthy woman (**55**) with no evidence of associated conditions such as pernicious anaemia, achlorhydria, diabetes mellitus or other autoimmune condition.

A typical site for vitiligo is on the knees (**57**), and on the dorsum of the feet. Figure **56** shows vitiligo on the forearm and **58** on the chest area, where it may be confused with hyperpigmentation secondary to sunlight and with pityriasis versicolor (**767**).

55

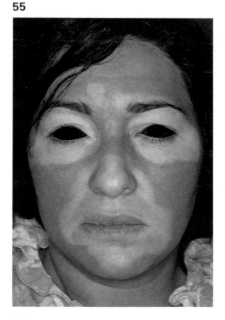

56

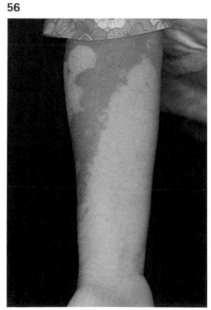

57

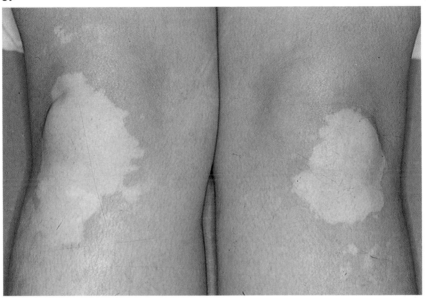

58

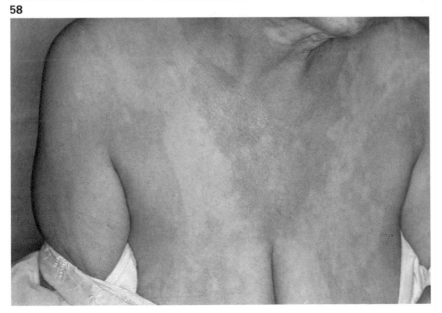

59 *Vitiligo* An early patch on the neck which may gradually enlarge. The hair pigmentation is unaffected. The depigmentation is due to damage to the melanocyte secondary to inflammation which may be autoimmune in origin and associated with other autoimmune disease, i.e. diabetes mellitus, Addison's disease (hypoadrenocorticalism), thyro-gastric disorders.

60 *Pityriasis versicolor* The flaking of the skin and apparent depigmentation after exposure to sunlight may mimic vitiligo but the characteristic distribution of the lesions in a peri-follicular manner distinguishes it. Once it becomes widespread it loses this peri-follicular distribution and can be a source of confusion to the inexperienced. Compare with **58**.

61 *Albinism* One has a complete lack of melanin due to the absence of a single enzyme concerned in tyrosine metabolism. Features are: (1) intolerance to sunlight; (2) white skin and hair; (3) pink iris; (4) impaired vision; (5) nystagmus.

62 *Heterochromia of the iris* A common failure of pigmentation of the eye, of no significance but sometimes disconcerting to the examiner and may be mimicked by the wearing of contact lenses!

59   **60**

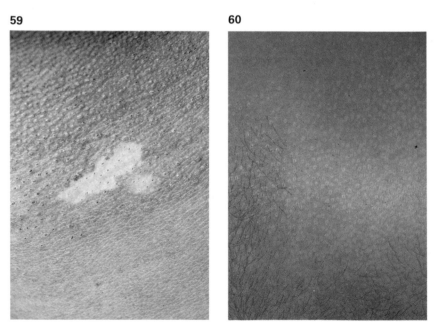

61

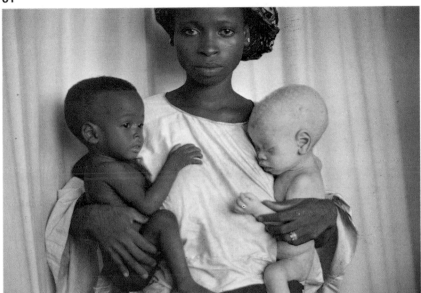

62

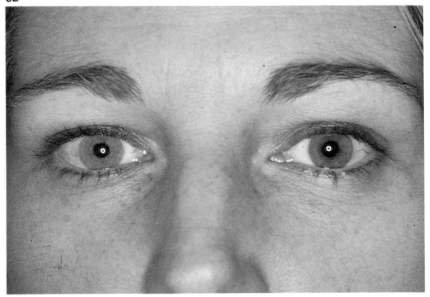

THE CLASSIC FACIES OF DISEASE

The classic facies of disease may superimpose themselves, overprinting the individual's own face. Even in their minor early forms they can be recognised by the trained eye and be the clue which can be grasped when the patient is first seen.

63–65 *Down's syndrome (mongolism)* The similarity is obvious in the baby, the toddler and the child of 12 years. (1) Eyes slope down to the midline, epicanthic folds prominent. (2) Nasal bridge is low. (3) The tongue is large and may be fissured transversely (**398**). (4) The hair is soft. (5) The hands are squat, a single transverse crease may be present and the little finger incurved (**489**). *(John Langdon Haydon Down, London Hospital, 1828–1896, described 1866.)*
   Compare these features with cretinism, **66**.

66 *Hypothyroidism (infant cretin)* The child is inactive and sluggish, pasty faced and constipated, the face coarse, the hair sparse, the skin cold, the tongue is large and he has a pot bellied abdomen, whereas the mongol is active, pink, the bowels normal.

63

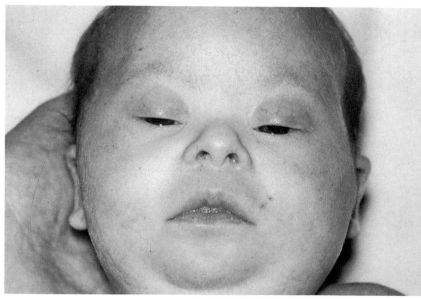

64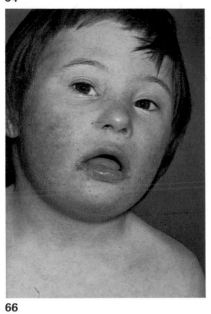

65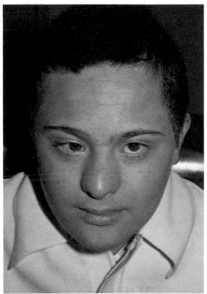

66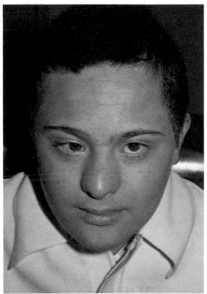

67 *Hypothyroidism (adult)* Myxoedema – appearance of the face in hypothyroidism is a summation of many changes which is often recognised at first sight of the patient as he walks into the room and if this association does not occur instantly it may be missed, particularly if the abnormality is minor. The apathetic look, pallor, thickness of the skin, dullness of the eye, broadening and podginess of the face, the thin hair, loss of eyebrows, coupled with the hoarse voice, slow speech and slow actions should suggest the diagnosis. Note the incidental corneal arcus, loss of hair on the temples, the fineness of the skin which is dry and the broadening of the cheeks with this 'myxoedematous look'.

68 *Myxoedema* The podgy face, a characteristic of myxoedema, is well seen here. Apart from this the thinness of the eyebrows is the only obvious abnormality and the diagnosis is suggested by clinical awareness rather than any specific point. Note the bilateral corneal arcus.

69 & 70 *Myxoedema* Lateral views of a man before and after treatment with Thyroxine.

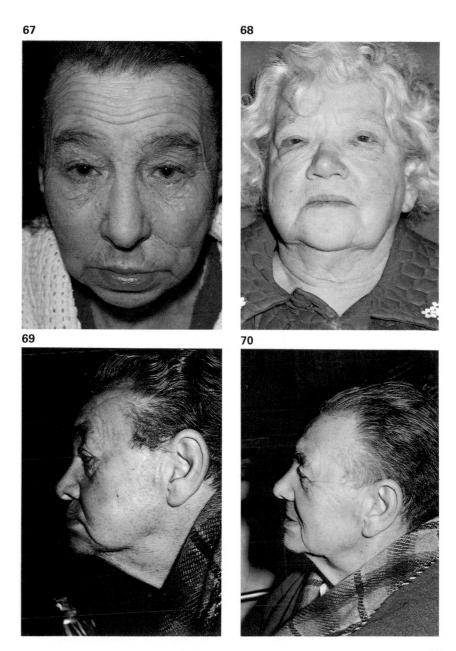

67

68

69

70

71-74 *Myxoedema* This woman (**71**) presented at a surgical clinic because of varicose veins and the surgeon recognised the condition as she walked through the door. She was directed to the medical department. The podgy, dull look, with dry, lifeless hair and the characteristic broadening of the lower part of the face is well seen.

After two weeks' treatment with Tri-iodo-thyronine (**72**) there is little change apart from a brightening of the eyes. Figure **73** shows the change after two months' treatment with Thyroxine. Most striking is the facial shape and the attitude. Five years later (**74**) shows thyrotoxicosis due to overtreatment!

71

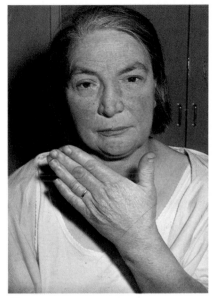

72

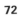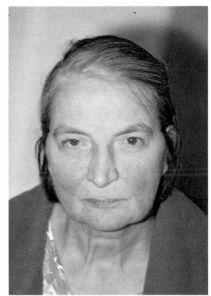

73

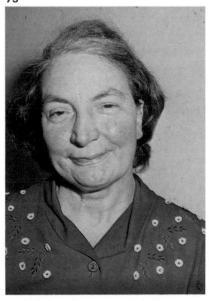

74

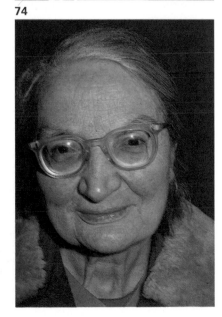

75 *Apparent hypothyroidism* Lateral view of woman with the facial suggestion of hypothyroidism and loss of hair at the eyebrow, puffy face and apathy, until she spoke, when she was bright and jolly. Her thyroid function studies were within normal limits.

76 & 77 *Borderline hypothyroidism* This man had mild hypothyroidism coupled with depressive illness. He has sparse eyebrows, a rounding of the face and presented with depression.

78 & 79 *Thyrotoxicosis* Before treatment (**78**). Note weight loss, tension, lid retraction more marked on the left, sweatiness of the skin. After two weeks' treatment with Carbimazole (**79**) there is a diminution in lid retraction, particularly in the left eye, and the tension appears to have gone out of the face.

75

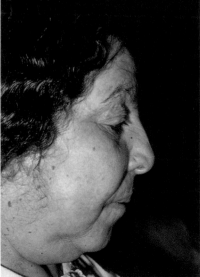

76

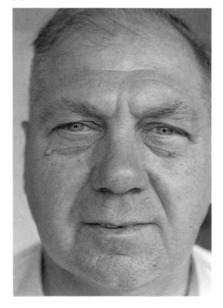

77

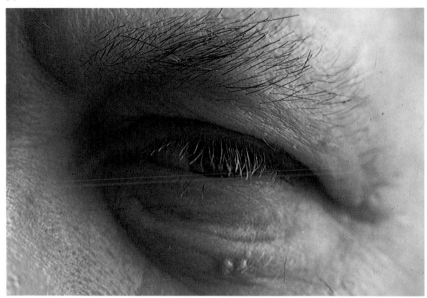

78

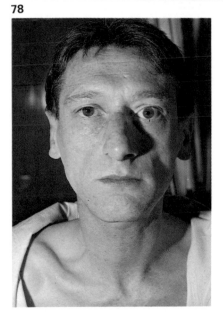

79

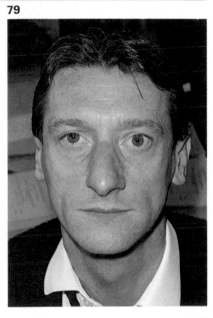

80–82 *Hyperthyroidism (thyrotoxicosis)* Note the tension in the face, the sweatiness of the skin, the exophthalmos and lid retraction of both eyes, more marked on the right eye (**80**). The white of the eye is exposed. Figure **81** shows the lid retraction and slight proptosis of the eye.

83 *Thyrotoxicosis (one month later)* After treatment with Carbimazole showing almost complete return to normal in the eyes, though there is still slight proptosis of the right eye. The skin is far less sweaty.

80

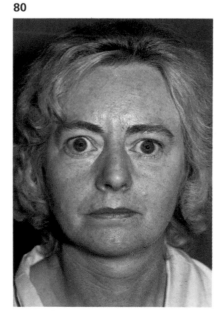

81

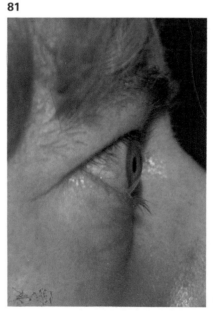

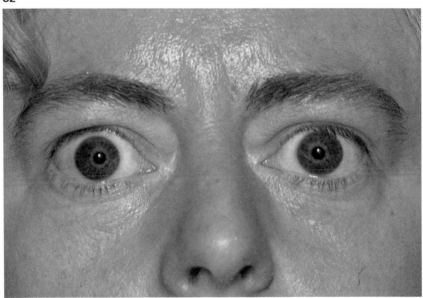

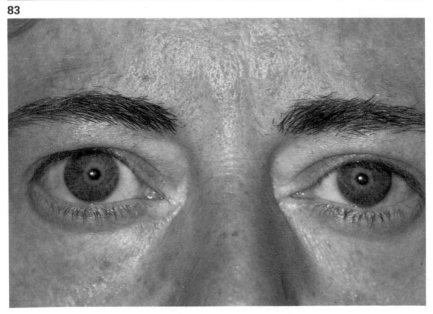

84 *Thyrotoxicosis* Bilateral lid retraction.

85 & 86 *Ophthalmic Graves' Disease* This man was euthyroid, but had thyroid auto antibodies and an elevated thyrotrophic stimulating hormone level. He subsequently became hypothyroid due to progressive Hashimoto's thyroiditis and developed progressive exophthalmoplegia: **86** was taken one year later. *(Robert James Graves, 1795–1853, described 1835.)*

87 & 88 *Thyrotoxicosis (middle aged)* This woman, 56 years, presented with recurrent attacks of explosive diarrhoea and weight loss. She was warm and sweaty with tremor of the outstretched hands and had a curious brown pigmentation of the skin.
　　The same woman (**88**) after treatment with Carbimazole and I^{131} showing weight gain, rounding of the face and loss of the tense look.

84

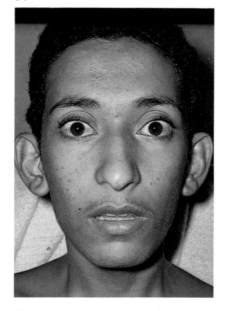

85

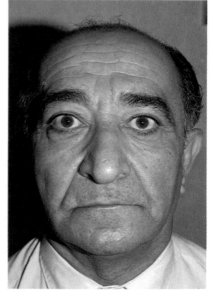

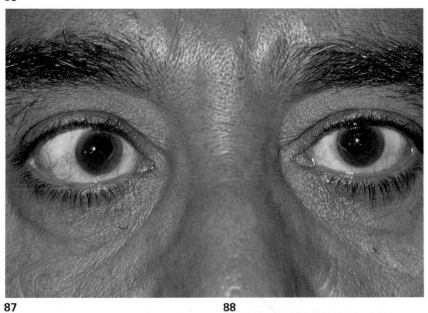

86

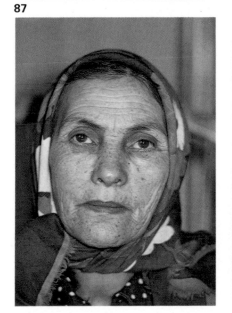

87

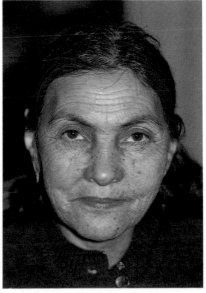

88

89–92 *Exophthalmos, thyrotoxicosis* The face has the tense look; lid retraction and proptosis are present and the lid cannot be opposed when the eyes are closed – early malignant exophthalmos.

93 & 94 *Malignant exophthalmos* This man had a three month story of weight loss, irritability and prominence of the eyes which had rapidly got worse so that the right eye developed corneal ulceration (covered), the left eye shows the gross lid retraction and exophthalmos. The cornea is already tending to dry because the lids do not sweep it adequately. This can be seen from the dryness of the light reflection on the cornea where the flash is reflected. In the lateral view note the proptosis of the eyeball and moist skin.

89

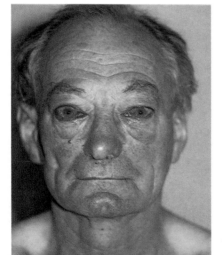

90

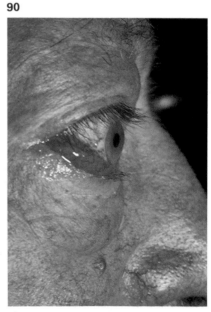

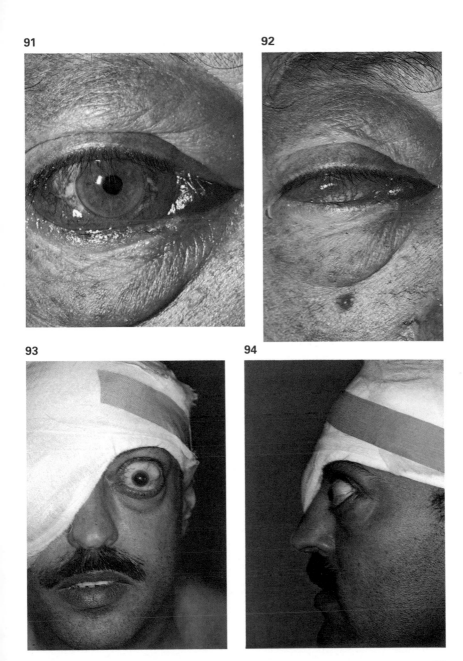

91

92

93

94

53

95 & 96 *Malignant exophthalmos* Thyrotoxicosis controlled with Carbimazole, the eyes had bilateral tarsorrhaphies performed.

97 *Obesity* The roundness and fatness of the face in obesity must be differentiated from the appearance of hyperadrenocorticalism (**98**).

98 & 99 *Cushing's syndrome* This young girl demonstrates all the facial features of hyperadrenocorticalism – Cushing's syndrome. She has a moon face with erythema and acne. Compare this with the photograph taken six months earlier, before the onset of her disease, which was due to a carcinoma of the adrenal gland. *(Harvey Williams Cushing, 1869–1939, described 1932.)*

100 *Cushing's syndrome, striae* In association with the mooning of the face, striae may be seen on the abdomen which characteristically are blue-pink in colour. These can be seen on this abdomen and on the upper thighs. This should be compared with striae gravidarum which occur in pregnancy and are white.

95

96

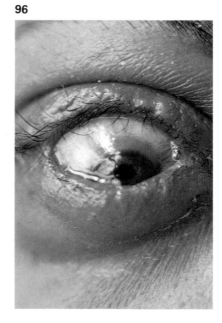

97 **98**

99 **100**

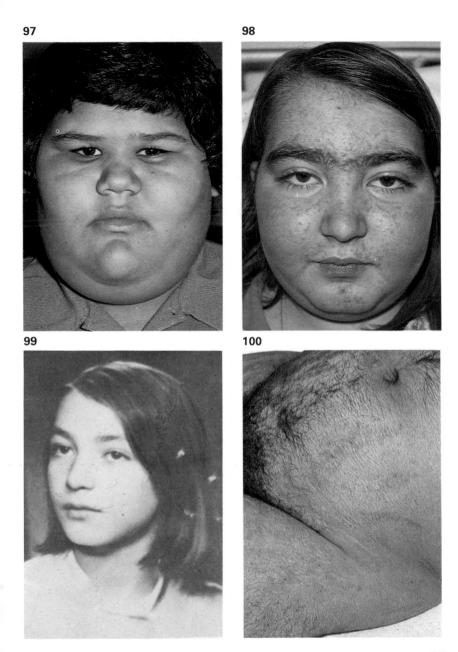

101 *Minor facial mooning*   The mooning of the face in Cushing's syndrome or following steroid therapy can be minor, as in this young boy with Behçet's syndrome (oral and genital ulceration) treated with steroids and it is this degree of early mooning of the face that should not be missed. The differential diagnosis of this physical sign is mild obesity; in both striae may be present but in the latter are usually pale and less livid. *(Halushi Behçet, 1889–1948, described 1937.)*

102 *Cushingoid facies*   The same child after nine months on high dose steroids for Behçet's syndrome with involvement of lung, heart, oral mucosa and scrotum. All the features of Cushing's syndrome are present.

103 & 104 *Cushing's syndrome (anterior and lateral view)*   Cushing's syndrome (secondary to steroid therapy) shows the deposition of body fat producing the characteristic 'orange on matchsticks' shape. Note the round, mooned face, malar flush, the striae over the abdomen and back and comparative slimness of the legs and buttocks with deposition of fat over the shoulders and upper back.

101

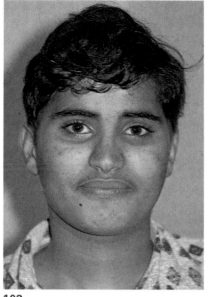

102

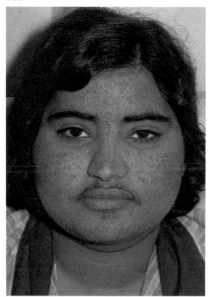

103

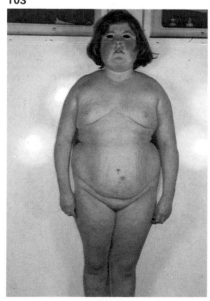

104

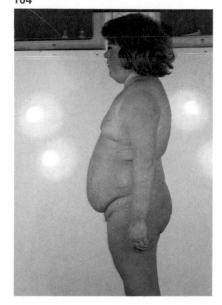

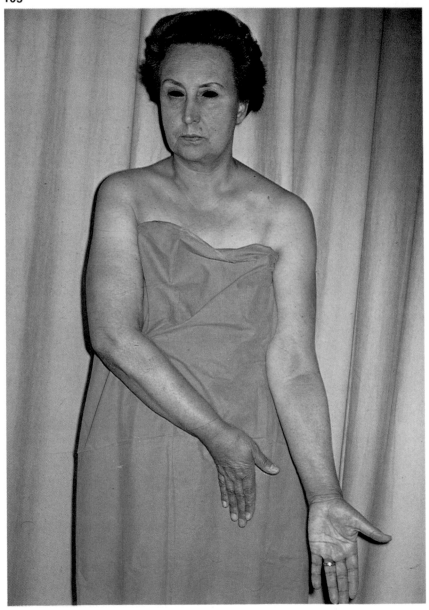

105 *Adrenocortical insufficiency* Addison's disease. May be primary due to adrenal gland destruction or secondary to pituitary/hypothalmic disease. Most cases of Addison's disease are either autoimmune or secondary to tuberculosis.

Acute insufficiency presents in stress situations on top of the chronic form – the classical physical signs being characteristically: (1) pigmentation of certain sites; (2) vitiligo – 15% of idiopathic Addison's disease.

Note the increased pigmentation of the hands, the palmar creases, the arms, face, shoulders and bra-strap area. *(Sir Thomas Addison, 1793–1860, described 1849.)*

106 & 107 *Addison's disease* In the European a characteristic pigmentation in the *creases of the hand* and on the pressure points of the body occurs. Differentiate this from the same appearance in the brown skinned races which is a racial characteristic – **107**, the palm of an Arab complaining of lethargy and suffering from depression, and which may be mimicked by henna on the palms.

106

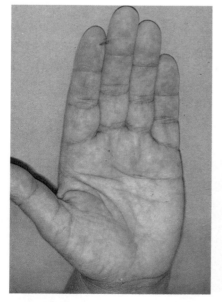

107

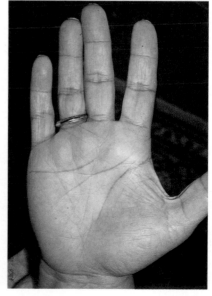

108 *Addisonian pigmentation* Pigmentation may occur in scars: here in the scar of an old varicose vein operation. All scars should be examined, the ones affected are those occurring after the onset of the condition.

109 *Addison's disease* Note the pigmentation of the gums.

110 & 111 *Addison's disease* Intra oral mucosal pigmentation in Addison's disease in a European, and similar pigmentation in an Arab on high dose tetracosactrin (synthetic ACTH).

108

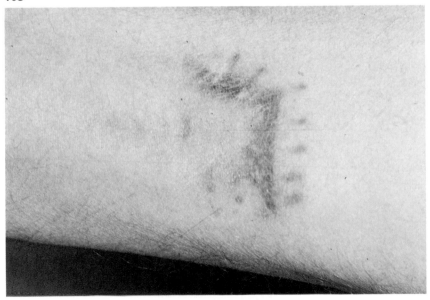

109

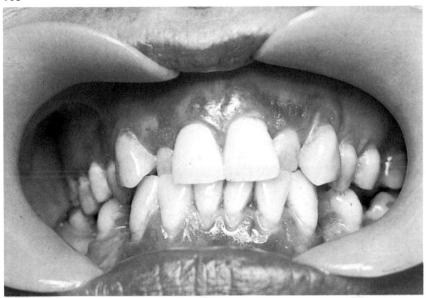

110

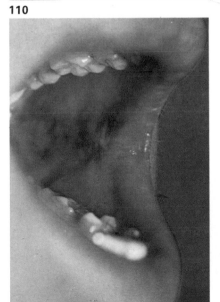

111

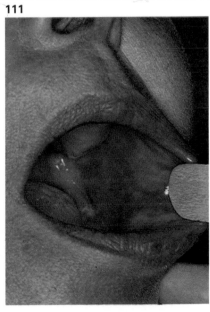

112–115 *Acromegaly* The coarse features, large nose, big tongue, spatulate fingers, secondary to a tumour of the pituitary producing an excess of growth hormone. This woman is of Middle Eastern origin. History: myalgia, paraesthesiae over a median nerve distribution of the hands, pains in the knees on walking. The face shows soft tissue thickening and a general coarseness of the features. Note the minor hirsutes. A nodule was felt in the right lobe of the thyroid gland – non toxic goitre is a feature of the acromegalic. In the lateral view note the increase of soft tissues, particularly of the nose, coarse features and the protuberant lower lip due to the increased growth of the mandible. As the patient swallows (**115**) the asymmetry of the neck can be seen, showing the goitre.

112

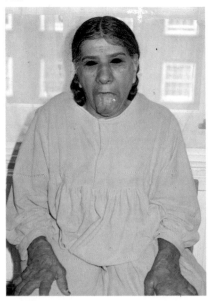

113

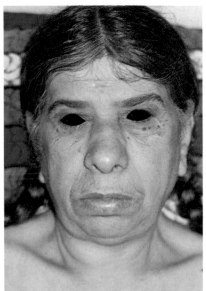

114

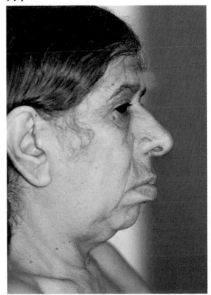

115

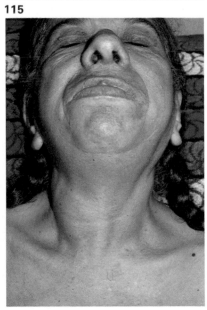

116–119 *Acromegaly* Now compare the next four pictures of a male acromegalic and note the family resemblance of the disease. The photographs show his driving licence 2 years before and his wedding picture one year before. The photographer deliberately made him turn and tilt his head to minimise the jaw. In the colour pictures note the big lower jaw, prominent orbital ridges and nose, and dramatic overbite due to the acquired prognathism.

116

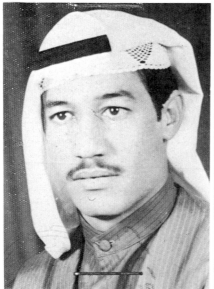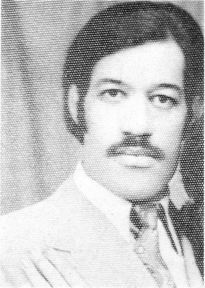

117

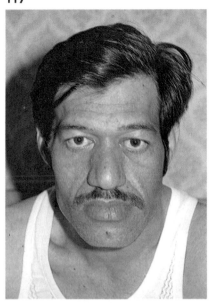

118

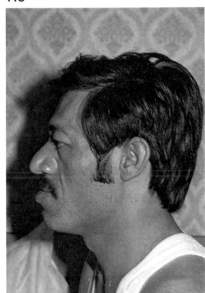

119

120 *Acromegaly* The lax skin secondary to soft tissue overgrowth on the forehead. One of the main problems was an increase in sweating which is associated with the increased growth hormone secretion.

121 *Acromegaly* The increased growth of the lower jaw takes the teeth forwards and they do not close in the bite correctly. This picture also shows the red line of gingivitis and pyorrhoea coupled with deposits of tartar which have become stained over the teeth. The hirsute upper lip is also seen.

122 *Acromegaly* With an increase in growth of the lower jaw the teeth become splayed and begin to separate.

123 *Acromegaly* The tongue may also hypertrophy, producing the appearance of macroglossia. Macroglossia must be distinguished from the large tongue which may occur in amyloid disease.

124 *Acromegaly* The normal large spatulate male hand above looks delicate beside the fingers of the acromegalic female. Note increase of soft tissues and broadening of the fingers.

120

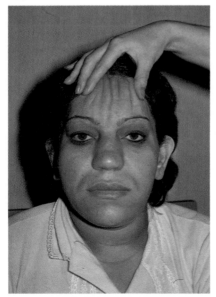

121

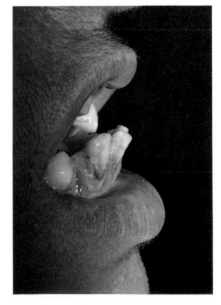

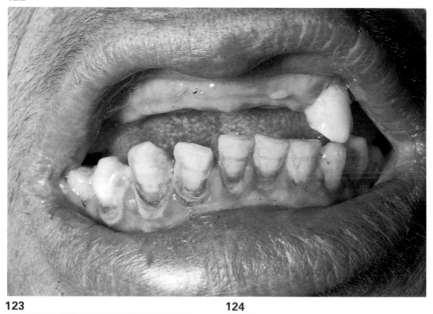

122

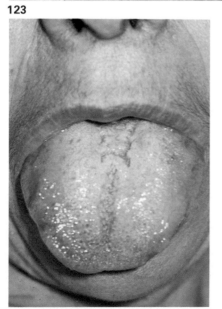

123

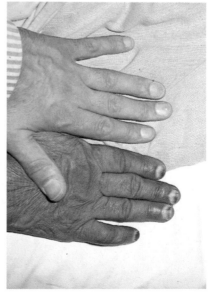

124

125 *Acromegaly (female)* The hands show the spade-like palm. Wasting of the thenar eminence is particularly obvious on the right hand, due to a carpal tunnel syndrome with median nerve compression.

126 *Acromegaly (male)* The soft tissue overgrowth is marked – on the left is the patient's brother, one year younger.

127 *Acromegalic feet* Note the increase in soft tissues and bony overgrowth causing the feet to increase in size and also to become broad and spade-like. Radiologically there is an increase in the cortical thickness with tufting of the terminal phalanx. All these signs are due to growth hormone excess.
Lactation had also continued for five years and the lactating nipple with very high prolactin levels is seen in **612**.

125

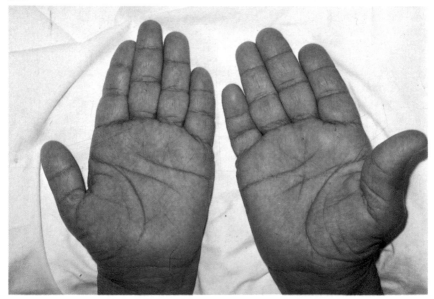

126

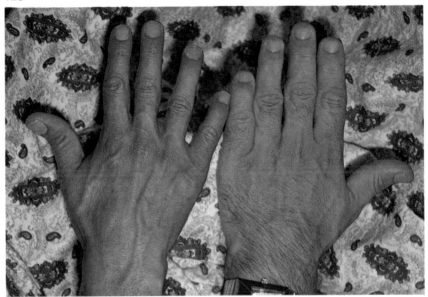

127

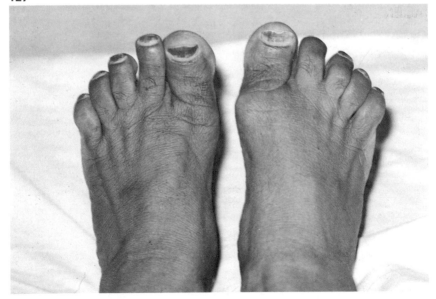

128–131 *Acromegaly – x-ray of hand* There is no great increase in joint cartilage but the early loss of concavity of the phalanges is well shown, particularly in the ring finger: minor tufting of the terminal phalanx is seen (**129**) and the balloon sella tursica (**130**) compared with a normal example (**131**) can be noted.

128

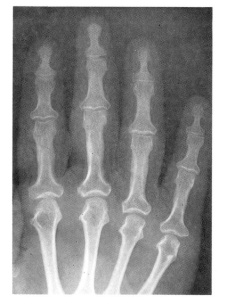

129

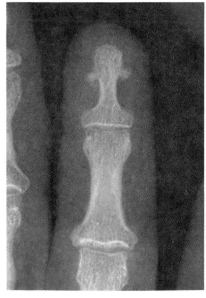

130

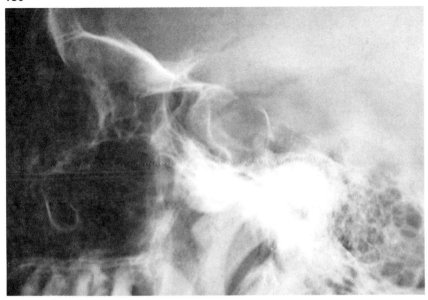

131

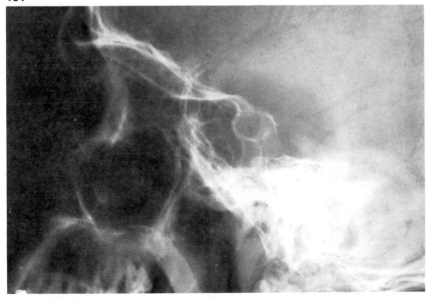

132 & 133 *Paget's disease* The increase in the size of the skull leads to prominence of the forehead.

134 *Paget's disease, x-ray* The x-ray appearance demonstrates the increase in thickness of the vault. *(Sir James Paget, surgeon, London, 1814–1899, described 1877.)*

135 *Paget's disease, bowing* A single bone may be involved. The thickened but soft bone bends: it may be warmer than the other due to increased vascularity. Bowing may occur in (1) Paget's disease; (2) Rickets – in 1 and 2 the soft bone bends; (3) Yaws, **691**; (4) Congenital syphilis – in 3 and 4 the bowing is more apparent than real as the long axis is unchanged.

136 *Sickle cell anaemia* The increase in the size of the skull due to thickening of the vault in Paget's disease should be compared to the similar thickening due to an increase in the medullary space which occurs in haemoglobinopathies. The similarity is obvious, the age group is different.

132

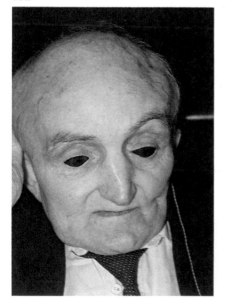

133

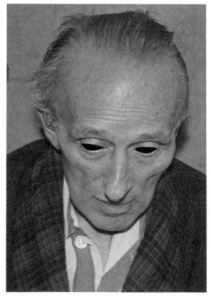

134

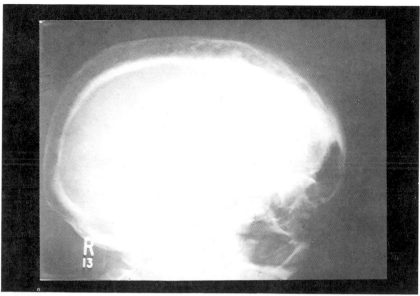

135

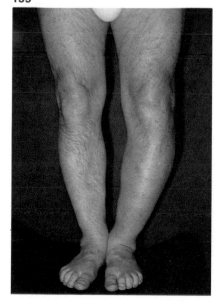

136

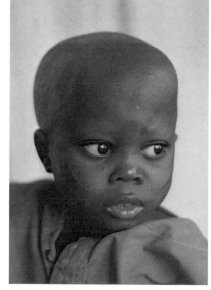

137 & 138 *Paralysis agitans (the shaking palsy)* The cardinal features are tremor, rigidity, and akinesia. A fixed flat expression devoid of emotion despite changes in circumstance, due to the immobility of the facial muscles. Note the sweaty, flushed look, from constant muscular activity. Patient **138** also dribbles excessively and finds swallowing requires effort. Because he tends to hold his head downwards in order to look at the camera he has to lift the eyes upwards – this is not the picture of an oculogyric crisis.

Oculogyric crisis, fixed upward deviation of the eyes, occurs in Parkinson's disease – post-encephalitic, phenothiazine overdosage, hysteria and hypoparathyroidism.

139 *Parkinson's disease* Stooped posture. The centre of gravity nearly outside the stable base, leading to a festinant gait – small steps always hurrying to keep the centre over the feet. Note abducted right shoulder and flexed elbows. *(James Parkinson, 1755–1824, described 1817.)*

137

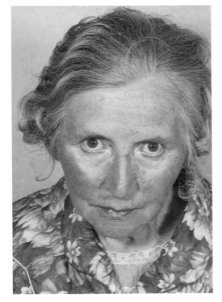

138

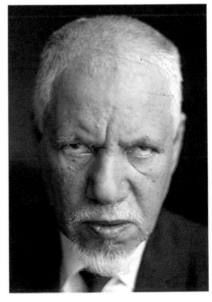

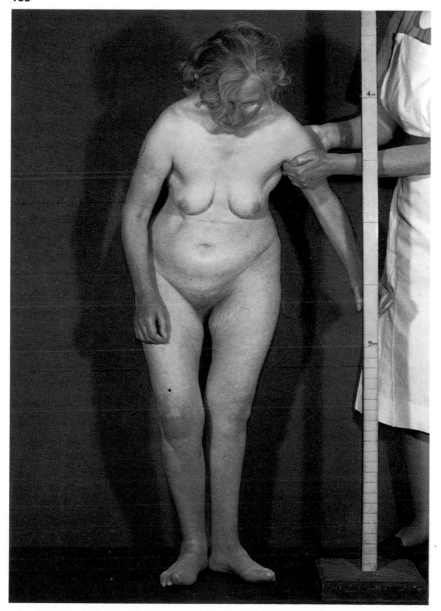

140–141 *Myotonia* Muscle tone may be increased in:

(1) extrapyramidal disorders, the tone is plastic in character with or without a 'cog wheel' component associated with tremor. The facial immobility of Parkinson's disease is due to the increase in muscle tone fixing the face.

(2) upper motor neurone defect – spasticity – clasp knife in character.

(3) myotonia – the muscle, once stimulated, remains contracted for varying periods of time and occurs in (a) Dystrophia myotonica; (b) Myotonica congenita (no dystrophy); (c) Paramyotonica congenita (increased with cold) (**141**). Myotonia may be spontaneous with voluntary effort (**142**) or demonstrated by percussion (**140**). This accounts for the delay in letting go on gripping something, particularly noted when shaking hands with the patient.

In this picture the triceps is tapped with a patellar hammer and a contraction of the muscle takes place which can be seen as an indentation running down from the shoulder. This persisted for three seconds, long enough to put the patellar down, pick up the camera and take the picture! The physical sign is brought out by cold surroundings, since the stiffness is always worse at a low temperature. In this particular patient he was perfectly well in the warm summer where he lived but noted the stiffness in the winter, and his children could not swim in the sea during the winter because they became very stiff.

140

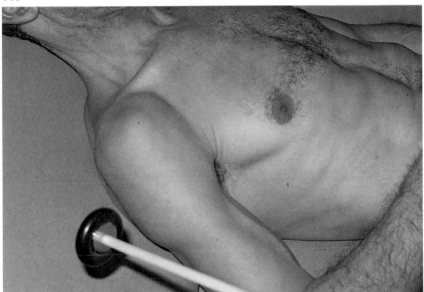

141

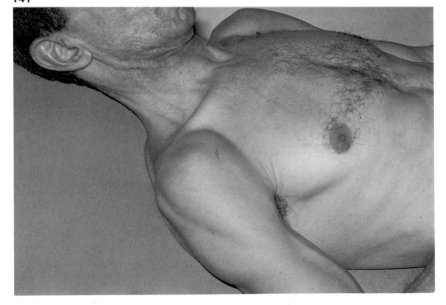

142–144 *Myotonia* These pictures show the sequence over four seconds when the patient was asked to squeeze the fist very hard and then open the hand VERY QUICKLY! It opens stiffly and in slow motion – the effort of opening almost shows.

142

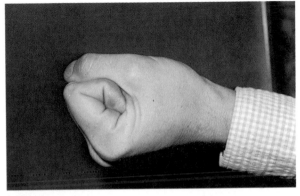

0 seconds (open quickly!)

143

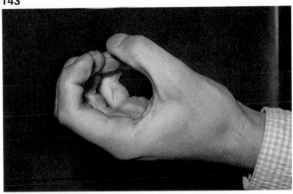

2 seconds

144

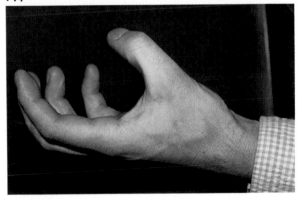

4 seconds

145–148 *Myotonia, lid lag* These pictures demonstrate lid lag due to myotonia of the eyelids. Look at me! (**145**). Look up! (**146**). Look down quickly! (**147** – the lid lags). Half a second later (**148**) the lid catches up and all is normal.

The same physical sign occurs in thyrotoxicosis but here the still camera can catch it as it happens in slow motion.

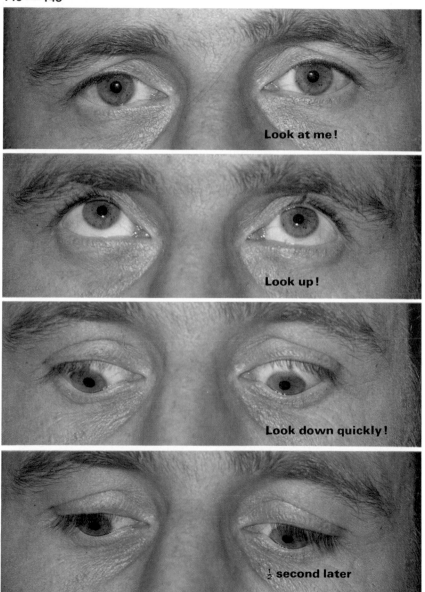

Look at me!

Look up!

Look down quickly!

½ second later

149–154 *Facial palsy, Bell's palsy* In repose it may appear that there is no abnormality present (**149, 150**). On closer appearance the face on the side of the palsy may have fewer lines, appear more youthful, and have less expression especially if the palsy is of long standing (**151**, forehead right).

Decide whether the palsy is unilateral or bilateral, upper motor neurone or lower motor neurone lesion at fault and if a lower motor neurone lesion, the site. The biggest catch is bilateral facial palsy (**153**). Ask the patient to smile (**154**). The commonest causes are acute infective polyneuritis, sarcoidosis, bilateral Bell's palsy.

The face is observed for symmetry, blinking, and examined by asking the patient to bare the teeth, close the eyes and then to screw up the eyes. Power is tested by trying to open them with the finger.

This young man has a mild right sided lower neurone lesion of the facial nerve (**149**). Asking him to screw up the eyes and show the teeth (**152**) results in an upheaval of movement of the face, pulling it to the normal side, often producing a momentary confusion in the inexperienced examiner's mind that it is the left side of the face that is at fault. *(Sir Charles Bell, 1774–1842, described 1821.)*

149

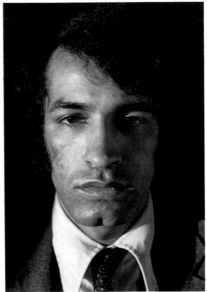

150

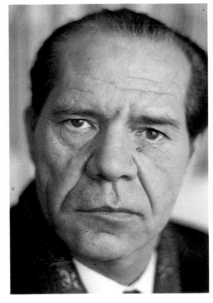

151

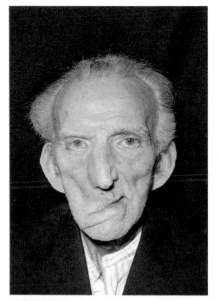

152

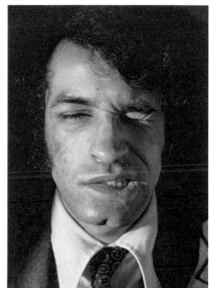

153

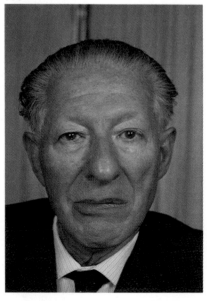

154

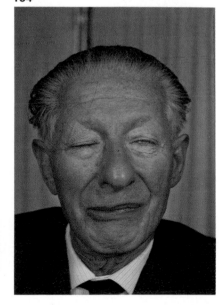

155–158 *Upper motor neurone lesion facial weakness* The weakness is predominantly of the lower face because the forehead is bilaterally ennervated. It is due to a lesion above the facial nucleus.

This man had a mild right sided hemiplegia due to a cerebro-vascular accident, (**155**, at rest). All that can be seen is a slight droop to the corner of the mouth on the right. Note the early corneal arcus. When asked to show his teeth (**156**) both sides of the mouth moved but the left moves much better than the right, and when asked to try harder and to screw the eyes up at the same time (**157**) it is seen that he has no weakness of the upper face, minimal weakness of the right lower face and weakness of the right platysma – the platysma is in action on the left side but not on the right. In contrast the emotional act of smiling (**158**) produces a much more normal movement of the face.

155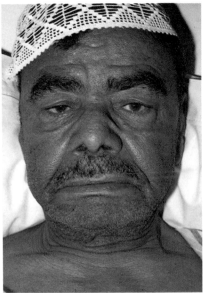

156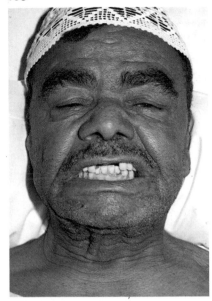

157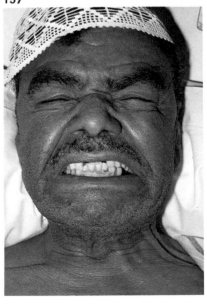

158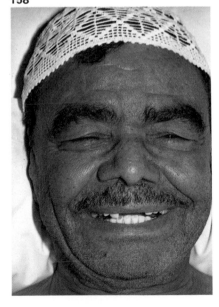

159 & 160 *Upper motor neurone lesion facial weakness of the tongue*
When asked to put out the tongue mild asymmetry is noted with slight deviation to the right side due to a right sided weakness of the tongue. Best seen in the close-up view – **160**.

161 *Unilateral lower motor neurone palsy* If the lesion is in the lower motor neurone there is total weakness of the face (**161**, 'raise your eyebrows'). The lesion is of the nucleus or more commonly the nerve.
Localise by:

(1) Herpes vesicles in the ear (**162**). The Ramsay Hunt syndrome due to involvement of the geniculate ganglion with the herpes virus.

(2) Any associated deafness, due to nerve involvement, points to a lesion in the cerebello pontine angle or in the brain stem. Conductive deafness may be unrelated or may indicate a lesion at the base of the skull such as a nasopharyngeal carcinoma.

(3) Loss of sensation of the 5th nerve points to a lesion of the brain stem or cerebello pontine angle.

(4) Loss of taste sensation on the anterior two-thirds of the tongue indicates a disturbance between the brain stem and the chorda tympani.

Other causes are: idiopathic or in association with diabetes mellitus; infections, tetanus and polio may present with facial palsy. Bilateral palsy (**153, 154**) occurs in sarcoidosis and acute infective polyneuritis and must be differentiated from myaesthenic weakness responding to edrophonium, and myopathic facial weakness (**257**). *(James Ramsay Hunt, 1872–1937, described 1907.)*

162 *Herpes vesicles in the ear*

159

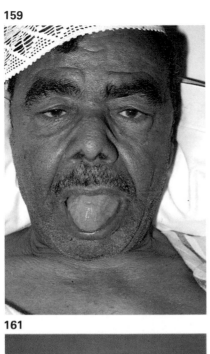

160

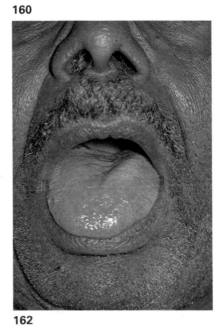

161

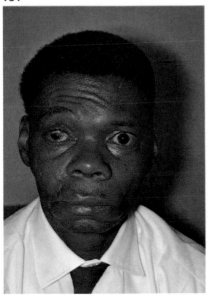

162

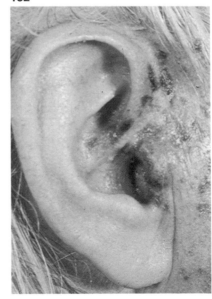

163 *Acoustic neuroma* Note: (1) tarsorrhaphy on the right (no corneal sensation); (2) lower motor neurone facial palsy on right; (3) he was deaf in the right ear for many years:

164–167 *Trigeminal neuroma* Complete fifth nerve palsy. Neurofibroma removed one year ago. Note: masseter wasted; temporalis – absent on the left side; left corneal reflex absent; the slight conjunctival injection; paralysed pterygoids – 'open your mouth'. May present as a cerebello-pontine angle tumour.

168 *Tabes dorsalis* The face in tabes. Note the loss of expression and the bilateral ptosis. Bilateral pterygia are present.

163

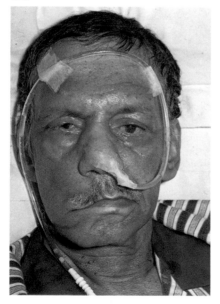

164

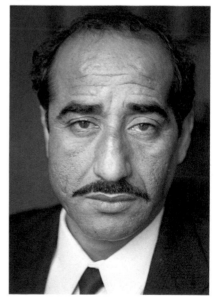

165

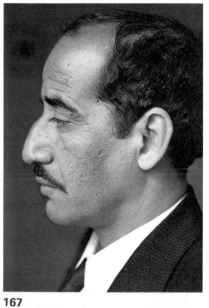

166

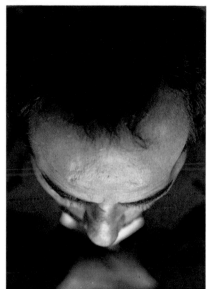

167

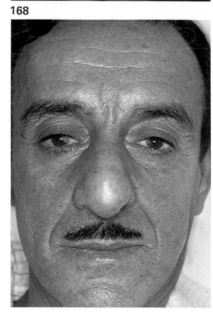

168

169 *Tetanus* This adult cut her foot and developed tetanus. The tension of the sterno-mastoids can be seen. Immediately after this picture was taken a door slammed and she developed a tetanic spasm with the classic risus sardonicus (**171**).

170 *Tetanus* This woman presented with stiffness. Note the tense sterno-mastoids as she sat waiting for consultation.

171 *Risus sardonicus*

169

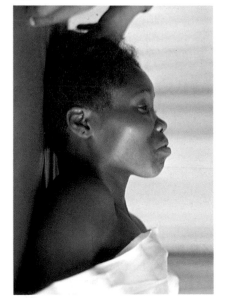

170

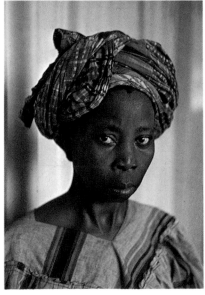

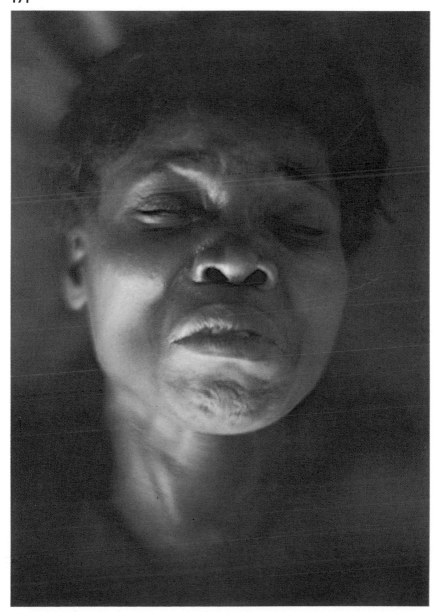

172 *Neo-natal tetanus with risus sardonicus* This form is usually related to cord sepsis and the practice of applying earth and cow dung to the cut umbilical cord. (See **636**).

173 *Lepromatous leprosy* The classical thickened skin on the ear and nose. The leonine appearance produced by thickening of the brows, note the loss of the eyebrows. The ear lobes present the appearance of a lepromatous infiltrate, the lesions being soft and succulent in appearance. They may be full of lepra bacilli and contrast with the well defined, clear cut margin of the tuberculoid type of leprosy. Between lepromatous leprosy and tuberculoid leprosy there is a continuously varying spectrum of disease.

174 *Lepromatous leprosy* The hypopigmented macules seen on this man's face are an occasional accompaniment of lepromatous leprosy when they occur early and are multiple, as opposed to tuberculoid leprosy in which they tend to be sparse.

175 & 176 *Lepromatous leprosy* These are examples of the skin lesions in lepromatous leprosy, with macule formation in the skin, lepromatous erythematous papules and associated raised and patchy areas of depigmentation.

172

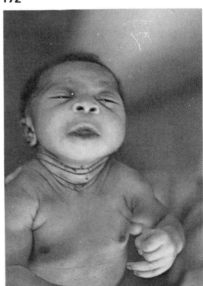

173

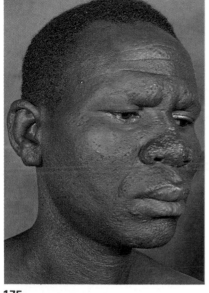

174

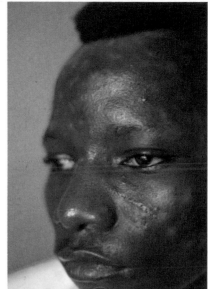

175

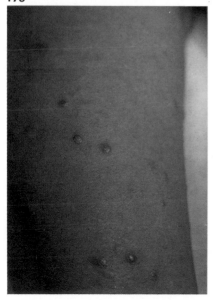

176

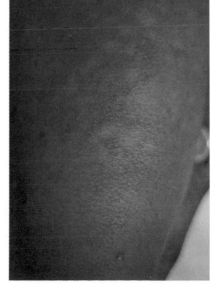

177 *Tuberculoid leprosy* Flat plaques of depigmentation, sometimes anaesthetic, may be the only skin change present. This is known as a macular-tuberculoid lesion compared with the lesion on the arm (**179**) which is a minor-tuberculoid with the one on the leg a major tuberculoid example of macular anaesthetic leprosy.

178 *Tuberculoid leprosy* The unnamed cutaneous nerves may be thickened and felt. The shininess is due to liquid paraffin spread on the skin in order to produce a light reflex and show up the bulge of the nerve running diagonally just above the ring finger extensor tendon.

179 *Tuberculoid leprosy* Benign, stable, presenting with skin lesions, associated with nerve involvement, often extending through cutaneous nerves. Plaques with red raised edges on the inside of the knee and forearm were insensitive to pinprick. The plaques spread slowly and were associated with some thickening of the peripheral nerves. The lepromin test was positive. The patient had been diagnosed as an example of sarcoid of the skin. The erythematous early lesion on the upper arm and the transition to the plaque can be seen in the lower lesion on the arm with a fully developed plaque on the leg.

177

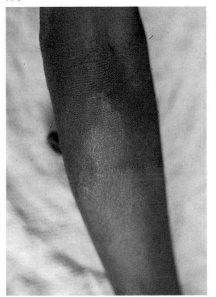

178

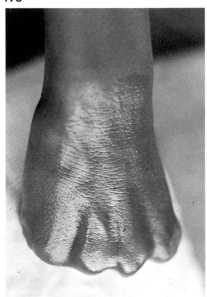

179

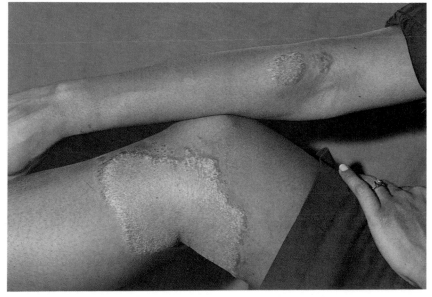

180 *Tuberculoid leprosy, thickening of the greater auricular nerve* This and figure **713**, a perforating ulcer, are all from the same patient.

The nerves should all be palpated for thickening: particularly the greater auricular where it crosses the sterno mastoid muscle, the ulnar nerve at the elbow, and the lateral peroneal around the fibula. The cardinal sign is one of anaesthesia. The sense of touch may be preserved but temperature and pain sensation lost.

181 *Tuberculoid leprosy* The thickened greater auricular nerve in the neck comes out from behind the posterior border of the sternomastoid and passes to the postauricular region. It must not be confused with a dilated external jugular venous system. Other causes of thickened nerves are: *congenital* – hypertrophic interstitial neuritis, neurofibromatosis; *traumatic* – repeated trauma to the nerve where it is exposed, e.g. at the elbow; *inflammatory infiltrations* – leprosy, sarcoid, amyloidosis; *neoplastic* – reticulosis.

Do not forget that in the thin and wasted person normal nerves may be palpable and may appear thickened. (1) greater occipital, (2) lesser occipital, (3) third occipital, (4) greater auricular, (5) nerves to levator scapulae, (6) accessory nerve, (7) medial supra clavicular nerve, (8) nerves to levator scapulae, (9) anterior cutaneous nerve of the neck, (10) cervical branch of facial.

180

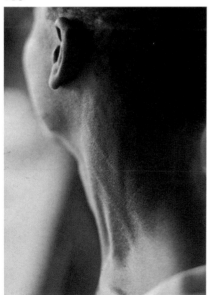

181

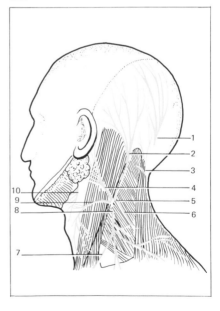

Facial skin abnormalities

Distribution of rashes on the face can sometimes allow a spot diagnosis. There are three kinds of Lupus – all unrelated: (a) lupus erythematosus, autoimmune; (b) lupus vulgaris, tuberculous; (c) lupus pernio, sarcoid granuloma.

Lupus erythematosus (LE)

A varying picture whose common factor is an increase of rash over areas catching the sun – the forehead, the malar bone and bridge of the nose.

(1) The classic butterfly rash, with or without plugging of pores, distribution related to light exposure. It has some similarities in distribution to rosacea but without pustule formation.

(2) A generalised erythema often increased over the face with oedema of the skin analogous to a severe sunburn. Seen in acute systemic LE.

(3) A macular/papular rash greater on exposed areas seen in acute systemic LE.

(4) Red plaques active and spreading at the edge with central scarring and telangiectasia, with a predilection for the face, nasal bridge, ear and scalp. On hair-bearing skin, scarring may lead to alopecia. Seen in chronic discoid LE.

182 *Lupus erythematosus* ' . . . erythematous patches . . . arranged in tolerable symmetry . . . the batswing or butterfly is very fairly attained . . .' One of the earliest illustrations of LE taken from Jonathan Hutchinson's Archives of Surgery 1890: the redness over the cheeks and forehead spares the shaded hollows of the eyes (compare with **183**).

183 *Systemic lupus erythematosus* He presented with arthralgia and oedema, the batswing erythema is 'tolerably well attained', some forehead rash is present and there is plugging of the pores over the cheek. Slight mooning of the face is present (not yet on steroids).

184 *Lupus erythematosus* The classic bat or butterfly wing: note the peripheral scaling. Compare this with rosacea (**185**).

185 *Rosacea* The distribution is across the cheeks and nose, associated with erythema, telangiectasia, and pustule formation which is not seen in lupus erythematosus, and often associated with facial flushing, increased by alcohol.

186 *Lupus erythematosus* Marked erythema in the V of the dress: macular/papular on the face.

182

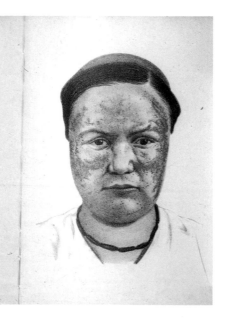

183

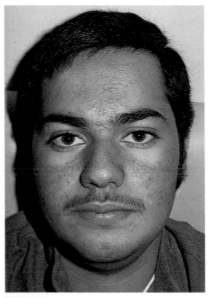

184

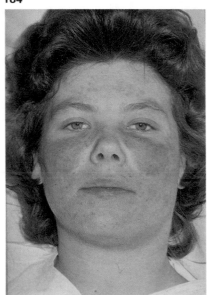

185

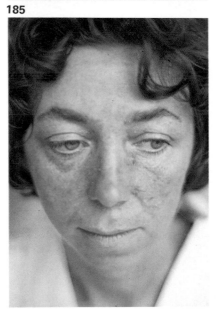

186

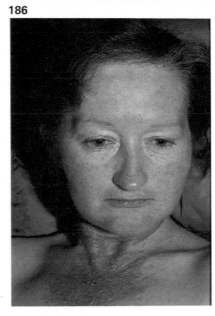

187 *Lupus erythematosus* Acute systemic illness, macular papular rash over the body increased on the arms, chest and face – sparing the area covered by short sleeves.

188 *Lupus erythematosus* Acute small joint arthralgia with pain and swelling of the proximal interphalangeal joints, part of the clinical presentation of the patient in **187**.

189 & 190 *Lupus erythematosus* There is slight facial oedema and erythema which blanches when the eyes are screwed up.

191 *Disseminated lupus erythematosus* This young girl has the erythema of butterfly distribution across the face. A nephritic facies of oedema – slit eyes – and the erythematous rash over the trunk, are sufficiently typical of lupus erythematosus to suggest the diagnosis. The facial oedema is typical of the so called 'nephritic' facies.

192 *Chronic discoid lupus erythematosus and TB gland* An area of scarring is seen over the bridge of the nose with depigmentation in the scar. There is no continuation of the rash over the malar areas and this example is confined to the bridge of the nose. Active red plaques are present in the.scalp.

187

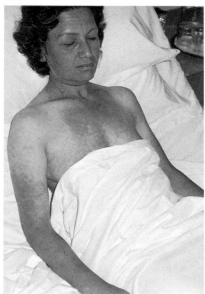

188

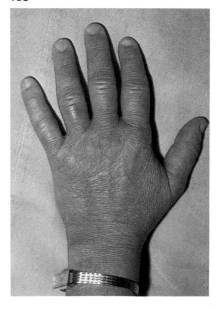

189

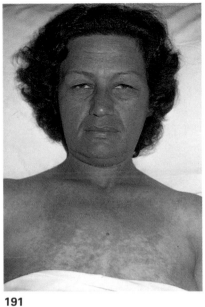

190

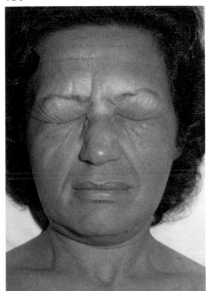

191

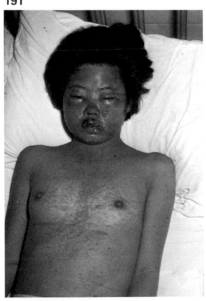

192

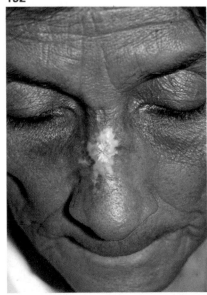

193 *Chronic discoid lupus erythematosus* In the scalp active red plaques can be seen. The central scarring on healing leads to alopecia.

194 & 195 *Chronic discoid lupus and TB gland in the neck* This woman exhibits two types of lupus. The scarring around the ear is healed Discoid LE while the reddening of the skin with the production of a sinus discharging pus seen in the supra clavicular area is typical of tuberculous lymphadenitis.

196 *Active lupus vulgaris (tuberculosis of the skin)* Exuberant hypertrophic ulceration spreading over the nose and malar areas.

193

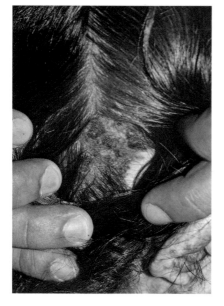

194

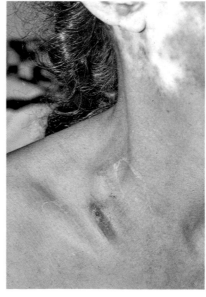

195

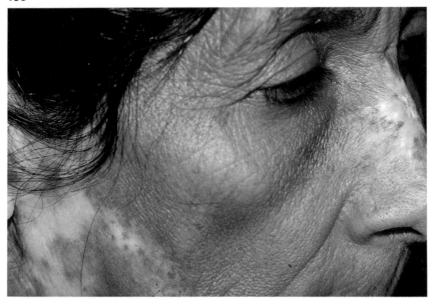

196

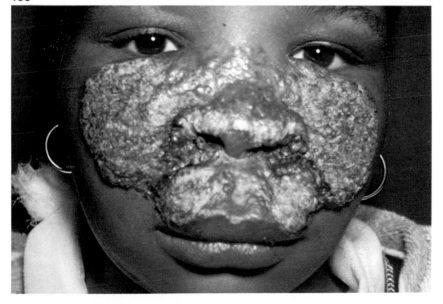

197 & 198 *Active lupus vulgaris* A less exuberant form which, when covered with a glass slide, exhibits the typical apple jelly appearance. This may progress to the situation shown in **199** with scarring and the destruction of cartilage.

199 & 200 *Inactive lupus vulgaris* In the healed stage scarring and destruction of cartilage, typically of the nose and the ear, occur. This lady had the 'new' treatment with the Finsen lamp (ultraviolet) in the early 20th century when the first lamp came to The London Hospital and to England.

197

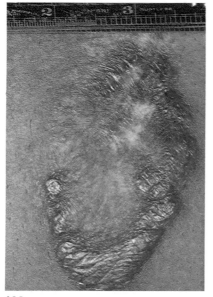

198

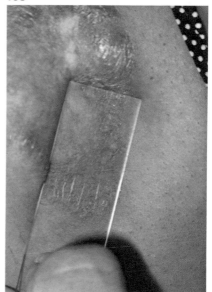

199

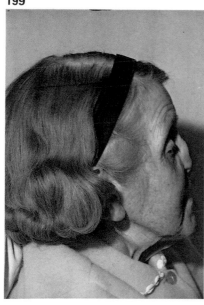

200

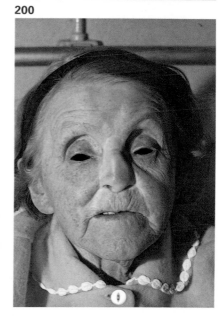

201–203 *Wegener's granuloma* An invasive granulomatous lesion affecting the nose and sinuses often presenting with lung lesions and a nephritis. It lies in a spectrum of disease between polyarteritis nodosa and lethal midline granuloma. This chest x-ray is that of a woman, the bridge of whose nose is destroyed in **201**. Note the solid lesions on her chest film, areas of granulomatous destruction and necrosis. Other causes of destruction of the cartilage of the nose are (1) lupus vulgaris, **200**, (2) leprosy and (3) tertiary granulomatous syphilis. *(F. Wegener, German, described 1939.)*

204 *Congenital syphilis (saddle nose)* Depression of the nasal bridge due to retarded growth of the septum and nasal bones due to persistent rhinitis in infancy. Compare with deformity in Wegener's granuloma when the nasal bones are involved with depression of the cartilage.

205 *Lupus pernio, sarcoidosis* This man shows red raised plaques on the right cheek and just below the nose. He has a facial palsy secondary to sarcoid – note the loss of small skin creases around the eye, the slight droop of the right side of the mouth and the normal skin creases on the other side.

201

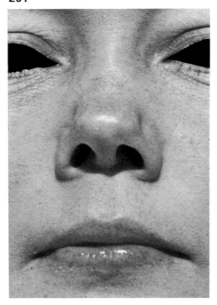

202

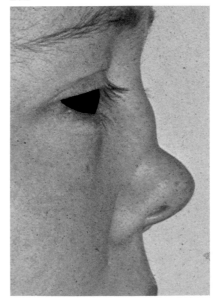

203

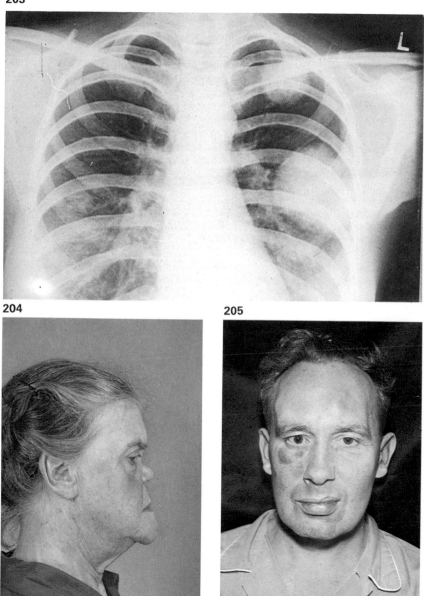

204

205

206–208 *Lupus pernio, sarcoidosis of the skin* Note the red, raised, bluish plaques of the skin which may be seen on the nose or face or isolated on the body. Skin sarcoid is often associated with bone cysts in the phalanges (x-ray).

209 *Facial oedema* The facial appearance is basically the same whether due to sodium and water retention in acute glomerulonephritis, hypo-albuminaemia in protein malnutrition, or local exudation in angioneurotic oedema, urticaria, allergy to insect stings and drugs, etc.

This woman presented with difficulty in climbing stairs and lightning pains. The WR was positive and the plantars extensor – she was treated with 14 days penicillin and steroids – at the end of the course and the cessation of steroids gross urticaria developed due to penicillin allergy originally suppressed by steroids. This subsided. The lightning pains remained and over the next six months the legs became weaker and the paraplegia more prominent – a myelogram, originally withheld, was performed and demonstrated a dorsal meningioma. *Double diagnosis:* neuro-syphilis and a spinal meningioma and not syphilitic arachnoiditis. *(Wassermann Reaction, August Paul von Wassermann, 1866–1925.)*

210 *Dermal wheals* The whealing produced after nettle stings and the exaggerated triple response of dermographism all produce transient dermal oedema.

206

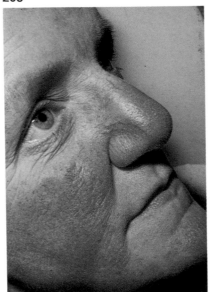

207

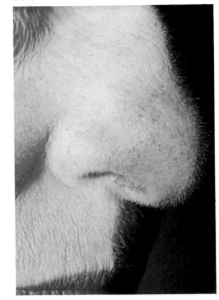

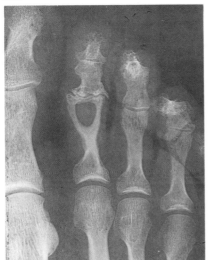

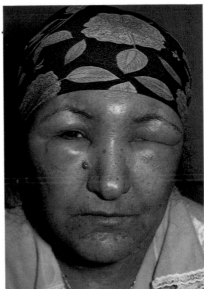

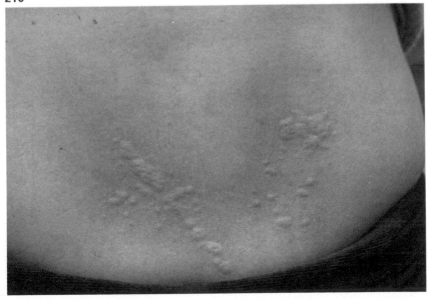

211 *Dermographism* This girl had recurrent attacks of urticaria with facial swelling – the initial blanching, flare and developing wheal are all shown.

212 *Acne vulgaris* Excess secretion of sebum and follicular inflammation – a problem of adolescence – the seborrhoea gives rise to a greasy skin and comedones (blackheads).

213 *Cystic acne vulgaris* The cysts contain pus – note blackheads and follicular inflammation.

214 *Sturge-Weber syndrome* Epilepsy and a capillary naevus in the ophthalmic division of the trigeminal nerve: there is an associated ipsilateral capillary haemangioma of the meninges often with cortical atrophy and calcification underlying it (which may be seen on plain x-ray).

One complication of the Sturge-Weber syndrome is epilepsy. In this case he was on Phenytoin which aggravated his acne. *(William Allen Sturge, 1850–1919, described 1879; Frederick Parkes Weber 1863–1962, described 1922.)*

211

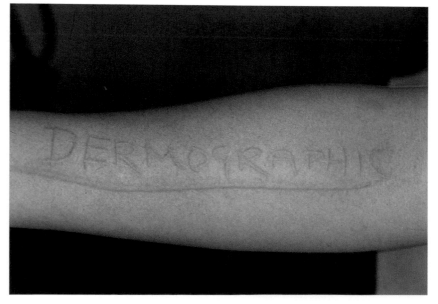

212

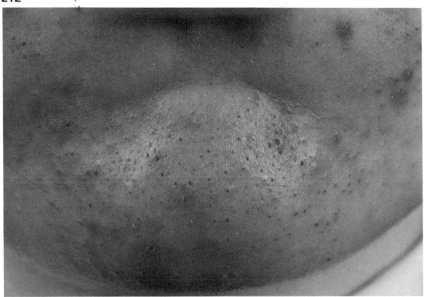

213

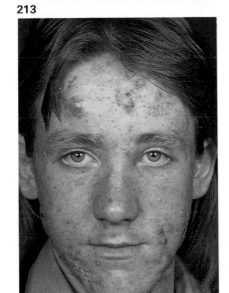

214

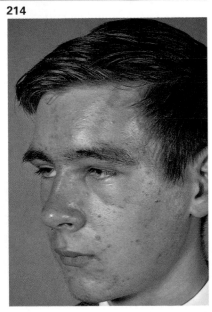

The hair

215 & 216 *The female hairline* Note that it goes straight across without the recession at the temples – this woman also demonstrated bilateral parotid enlargement due to sarcoidosis.

217 & 218 *Recession, male and female* The typical male temporal recession. This man also has a cautery mark on the forehead done in childhood in the Middle East. The frontal recession seen typically in the male differs in its form from the widow's peak hair recession in females, seen here in this woman who also has a well marked chloasma.

219 *Widow's peak, male* A similar appearance may be seen in the male with a widow's peak phenomenon, a female hair line and Klinefelter's syndrome, the chromosomes being XXY.

215

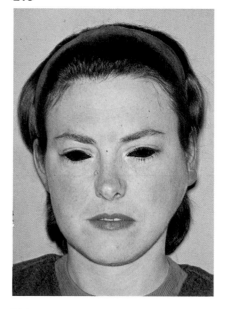

216

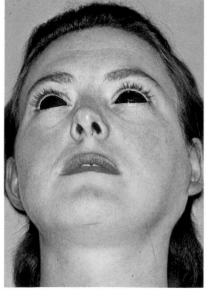

217

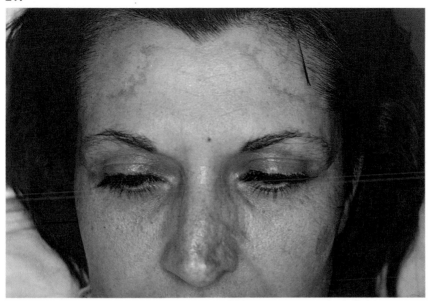

218

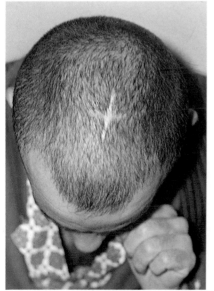

219

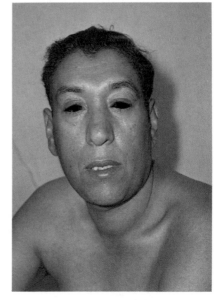

220 *Recession and psoriasis* The normal male temporal recession of hair in a man with psoriasis of the scalp.

221 *Recession in progress* This temporal recession progresses with a gradual loss of hair over the frontal area as in this man who also demonstrates the increase in the size of the skull secondary to Paget's disease (osteitis deformans). *(Sir James Paget, 1814–1822, described 1877.)*

222 *Complete top recession* The typical frontal baldness of the male may progress until hair over the top of the head is completely lost whilst a normal growth continues at the sides and back.

220

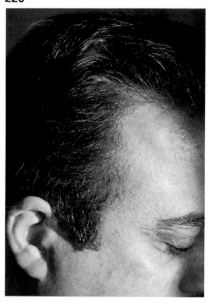

221

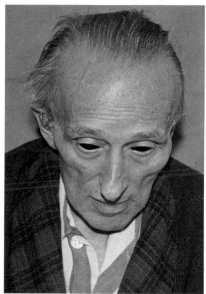

222

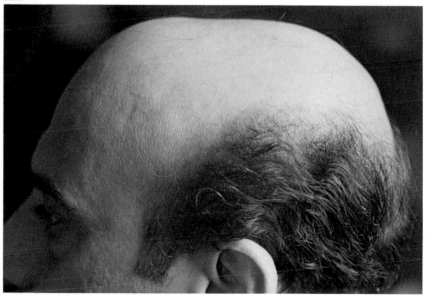

223–225 *Alopecia areata* Patchy loss of hair may be due to alopecia areata which may affect the scalp (**223**), eyebrows, eyelashes (**224**) and is of unknown origin. Exclamation mark shaped hairs may be seen. Hair may regrow with depigmentation or total loss may occur progressing to alopecia totalis. Temporal hair loss may also be related to pulling on the hair, in Western Society the pigtail and in Africa the continual pulling on the hair to produce various hair styles as in **225**. This girl also demonstrated keloid formation in the ear lobe following ear piercing.

223

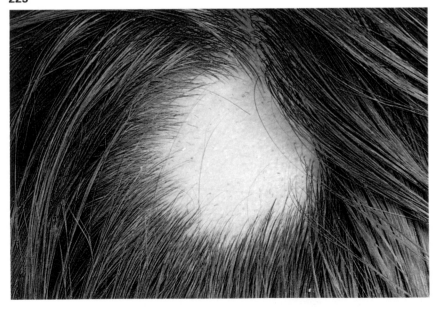

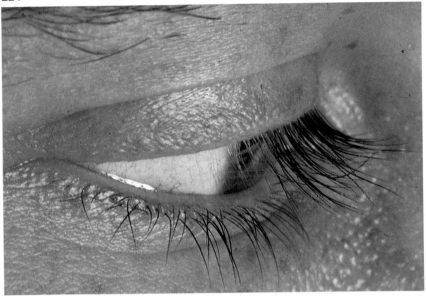

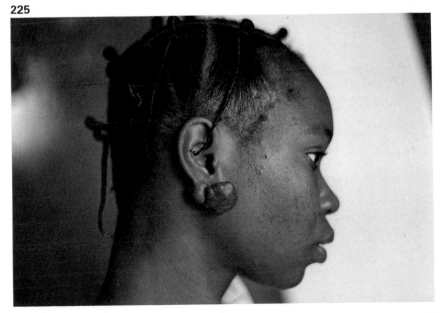

226 *Malnutrition baldness* Severe malnutrition may lead to depigmentation of the hair and sparseness as seen in this woman with malnutrition secondary to tuberculosis.

227 *Baldness secondary to x-ray epilation* Regrowth is beginning after this ringworm treatment.

228 *Scarring alopecia (LE)* The plaques of chronic discoid lupus erythematosus scar and lead to baldness.

Other miscellaneous conditions

229 *Scleroderma* The shiny, tight skin of the hands and the atrophic nails with disorder of nail growth are typical of systemic sclerosis. There is patchy telangiectasia of the face.

226

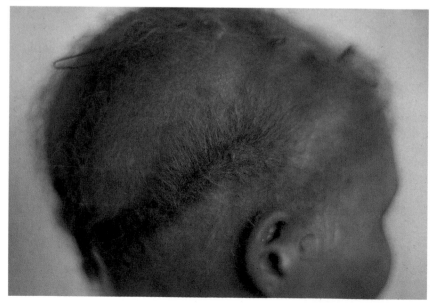

227

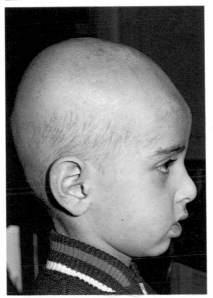

228

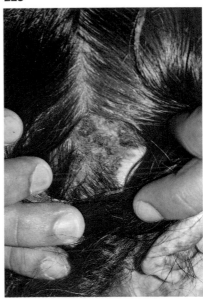

229

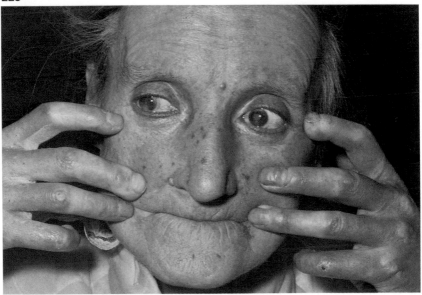

230 & 231 *Scleroderma* These hands show the shiny skin and should be compared with the previous slide. Here the changes are minor with slight firmness and shininess. The change is best appreciated by touch.

232 *Scleroderma* In this early case note the shiny inelastic quality of the skin under the chin and the numerous telangiectases.

233 *Scleroderma* As the disease progresses and the skin becomes tighter the face loses its normal wrinkles and expression. Many telangiectases.

234 & 235 *Local scleroderma (en bande)* Atrophy of subcutaneous tissue beneath the tethered and thickened skin (**234**). Note the patchy pigmentation over the upper arm. This variety of scleroderma is not associated with systemic manifestations.

230

231

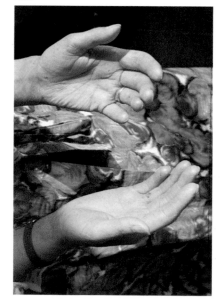

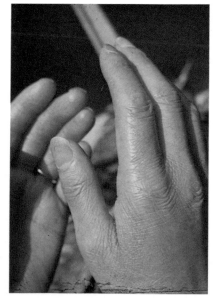

232

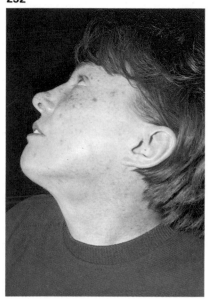

233

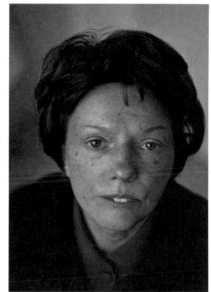

234

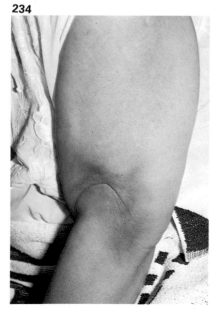

235

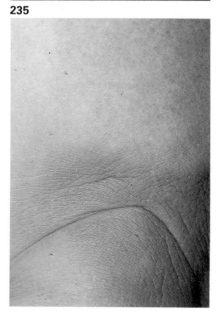

236 *Malar flush* The erythema across the cheekbones is by tradition associated with tight mitral stenosis. However you can see this in fit people of all walks of life whether they live in the open air or not. It is probably one of the traditional associations of medicine without foundation in fact.

237 *The febrile patient* This man is ill. He is hot, sweating, the eyes are slightly sunken and the face is apathetic. He has a lobar pneumonia, temperature 104°F (40°C).

238 *Fever and herpes simplex* Herpes febrialis – this woman had pneumonia and shortly after admission developed the patch of herpes on the upper lip. A characteristic association with fever.

239 *Herpes genitalis (simplex)* Herpes genitalis with intact vesicle and no crusting. Recurrent condition, common, often gives rise to unjustified alarm.

236

237

238

239

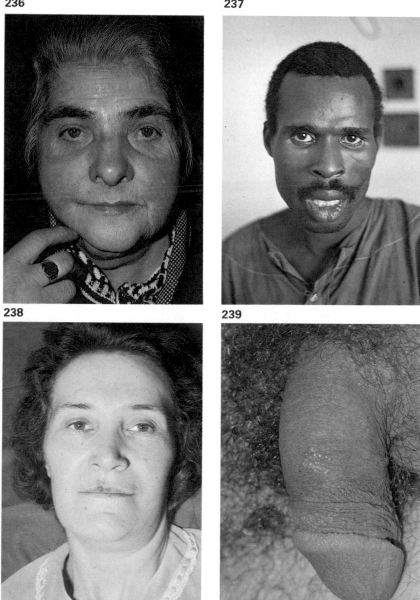

240 & 241 *Herpes zoster: early* The rash of herpes begins as a macule which developes into a vesicle on a red base in the distribution of the dermatome. The close-up study (**241**) shows the lesion which should be compared with the rash in the Negro where the erythema cannot be seen. The rash may be very sparse and the main complaint be of pain or paraesthesia in the distribution of the nerve.

242 & 243 *Herpes zoster (shingles), florid* This is distributed over one dermatome, stops at the midline, and affects half the umbilical hernia. Florid vesiculation is seen in the lateral view, following the dermatome.

240

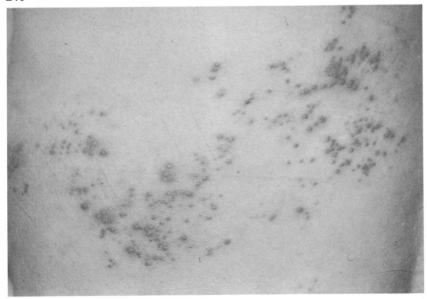

241

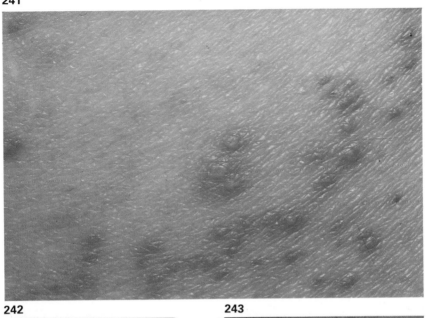

242

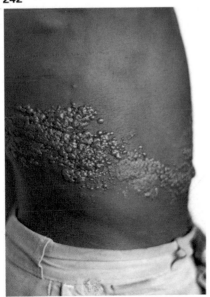

243

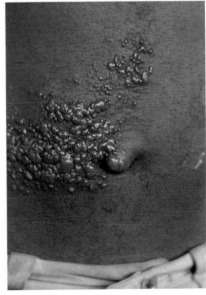

244 *Herpes zoster* The lesion progresses with rupture of the vesicles, crusting and then scarring, producing this end result on the trunk.

245 *Distribution of cutaneous nerves to head and neck*

246 *Herpes zoster (scarring)* Affecting the trigeminal nerve – ophthalmic branch. Here the residual scarring is seen extending into the hair but with no corneal scars. The midline is not crossed by the scars.

247 & 248 *Herpes zoster (Vth maxillary)* The appearance is due to the application of Calamine lotion to the lesion by the patient. The territory supplied by the maxillary division of the fifth cranial nerve is affected. Note the vesicles extending up between the eyebrows onto the forehead – the zygomatic – temporal branch of the zygomatic nerve, (a branch of the maxillary divisions of the Vth) has a variable temporal distribution.

244

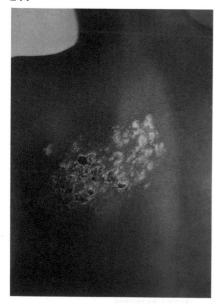

245

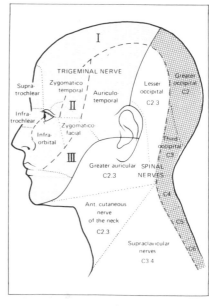

246

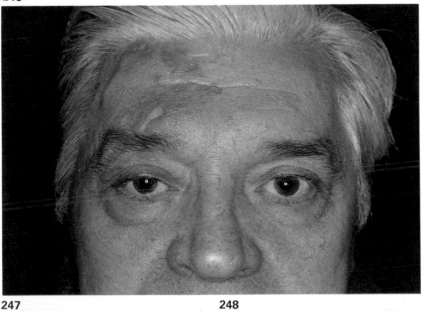

247

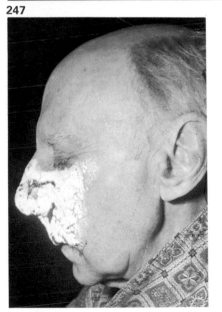

248

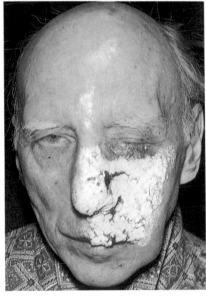

249 & 250 *Chloasma ('uterini' or 'bronzium')* This patchy pigmentation is seen on the face, either as a mask around the eyes or across the forehead. It may occur in pregnancy, and in women who are taking the contraceptive pill, particularly if they have been exposed to sunlight. The appearance may be mimicked by the pigmentation produced on the skin after the application of perfumes and exposure to sunlight.

249

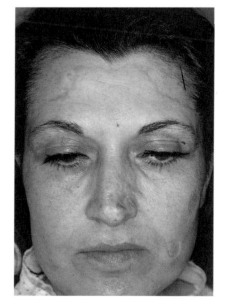

250

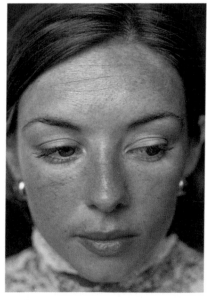

THE EYES

Ptosis or drooping of the eyelids (Ġk falling)

Ptosis may range from minimal droop to total closure. When confronted with unilateral ptosis, particularly if not severe, you must distinguish it from lid retraction of the other eye. Is it bilateral in fact, but asymmetrical? Is it associated with (1) an over reactive frontalis muscle (tabes) or is the over reaction on the opposite side from the ptosis (functional)? Or is it associated with (2) inequality of the pupils (Horner's or IIIrd nerve palsy) or with ocular palsy?

Causes of ptosis

Tabes dorsalis. Bilateral ptosis, bilateral frontalis overaction may be present.

Congenital. Bilateral, occasionally unilateral ptosis. Bilateral frontalis overaction may be present.

Myopathic. Dystrophia myotonica. Bilateral, with wasting of the face.

Myasthenic. Increasing with upward gaze. Bilateral or asymmetrical, partial or complete.

Sympathetic nerve lesion. Unilateral, partial, smaller pupil.

Oculomotor. IIIrd nerve lesion, unilateral, partial or complete, pupil larger, with a divergent squint (unopposed lateral rectus action).

Functional. Unilateral or bilateral, partial or complete, frontalis overaction on the *opposite* side, often associated with blepharospasm.

Miscellaneous. Drugs: bethanidine eye drops. Trauma/operation with longstanding occlusion.

251 *Bilateral ptosis, tabes dorsalis* This is usually bilateral, the face is expressionless and sad. Bilateral frontalis overaction may be present as well, giving a 'surprised' expression. No pupillary changes can be seen though there was a very sluggish reaction to light compared to the briskness on convergence. There is a pterygium in the right eye.

252 *Bilateral ptosis, tabes dorsalis* The man also has Argyll Robertson pupils, which can be seen in **253**. *(Douglas Moray Cooper Lamb Argyll Robertson, 1837–1909, described 1868, Edinburgh.)*

251

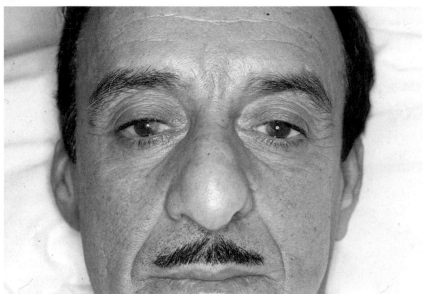

252

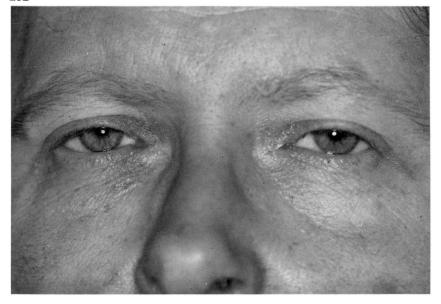

253 *Argyll Robertson pupil* Close-up of the pupil of the preceding photograph showing the irregularity of the pupil with some atrophy of the eye pigment adjacent to the pupil. The pupils are small, irregular, and unequal, and they react poorly to light and mydriatics and briskly on convergence, and have atrophic irides.

254 & 255 *Congenital ptosis* Usually bilateral but may be unilateral. Other associated abnormalities are congenital facial diplegia, external ophthalmoplegia, lingual palsy, or club foot.

253

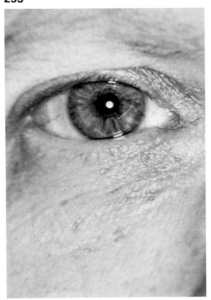

254

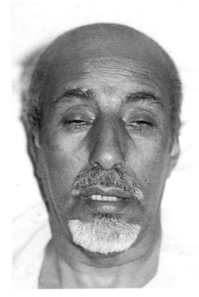

255

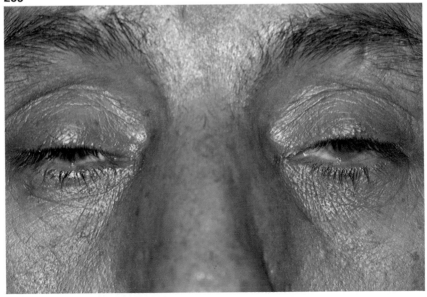

256 *Congenital ptosis* A left sided unilateral ptosis is present without frontalis overaction. It is nearly complete and there is no obvious squint suggesting that it is not due to a third nerve palsy. The pupil cannot be seen. Ptosis of this degree, if not due to a third nerve palsy or a sympathetic lesion could only be congenital since congenital ptosis can occur unilaterally. Myasthenic unilateral drooping is a serious differential diagnosis.

257 *Dystrophia myotonica* Bilateral ptosis is present with consequent extension of the neck and slight frontalis overaction to try to improve the vision. Early frontal baldness and atrophy of facial muscles are present. Sterno-mastoid weakness is present.

258 & 259 *Ptosis and myasthenia gravis* Bilateral ptosis is present, there is slight frontalis overaction. There is demonstrable fatiguability on upward gaze with increasing ptosis. There may be an accompanying ocular palsy and consequent diplopia. Note: myasthenic ptosis *may* be unilateral.

The intravenous injection of edrophonium chloride produces dramatic improvement but only lasting for one minute (**259**).

256

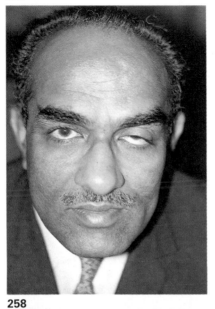

257

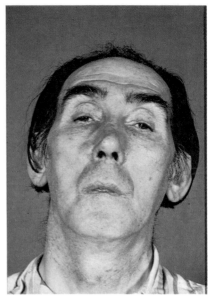

258

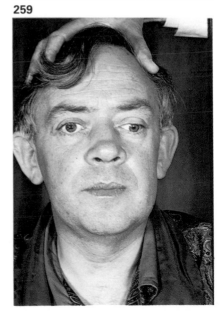

259

260–265 *Ptosis and myasthenia gravis* Unilateral, complete – superficially like a third nerve palsy. Thirty seconds after edrophonium chloride intravenously the ptosis is disappearing and the weak extraocular muscle can be seen: subsequently at twenty second intervals the effect of the injection wears off and complete ptosis returns. The tears are caused by the uncomfortable feeling and drain to the left nostril and also overflow down the cheek. Twenty seconds after **265** the boy appeared the same as in the first picture of the series.

260   0 seconds   **261**   30 seconds

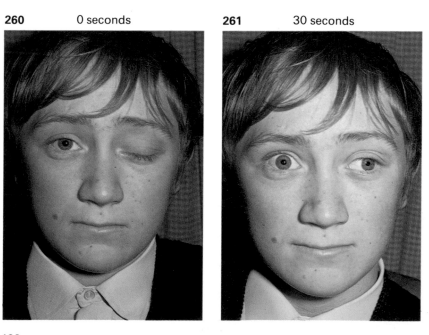

262

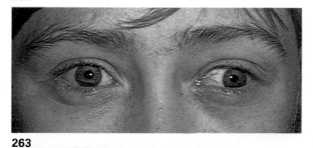

50 seconds

263

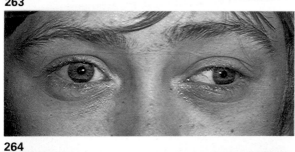

70 seconds

264

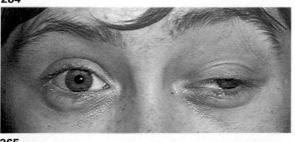

90 seconds

265

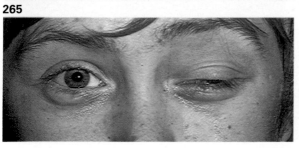

110 seconds

266 *Ptosis, cervical sympathetic lesion* A young girl with a right sided ptosis and trophic changes in the fingers. 'Deductive looking' would lead one to suggest that the finger could be due to a burn, gangrene, Raynaud's phenomenon, an embolus, ergotism or a cervical rib. The small pupil with a right sided ptosis were related. The lid of the right side definitely is ptosed since (1) there is overaction on the right, (2) there is a small pupil on the right, (3) the lid cuts tangentially across the small *and* the larger pupil – the right lid must be lower. Relating these two together we have a sympathetic nerve lesion of the eye with the finger change. Diagnosis is a cervical sympathectomy for a severe Raynaud's phenomenon. An alternative possibility is burns in syringomyelia. *(A G M Raynaud, 1834–1881, described 1862.)*

267–269 *Ptosis, Horner's syndrome* Partial ptosis is present on the right hand side with a smaller right pupil. The remainder of the syndrome – exophthalmos and defective sweating – is not seen. It is debatable whether exophthalmos is ever easily detectable. In this case the diagnosis becomes obvious with the presence of wasting of the small muscles of the hand (**269**). The thenar and hypothenar muscles are wasted (first thoracic segment). The lesion here was due to interruption of the sympathetic chain by an apical carcinoma of the lung (**268**), Pancoast tumour. *(Johann Friedrich Horner, 1831–1886, described 1869 with apical tumour; Henry Khunrath Pancoast, 1875–1939, described 1932.)*

266

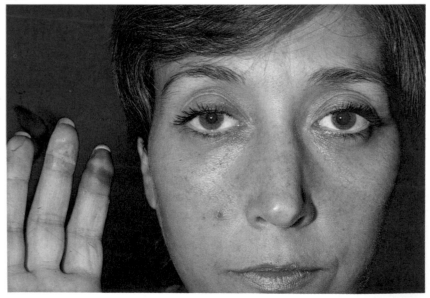

267

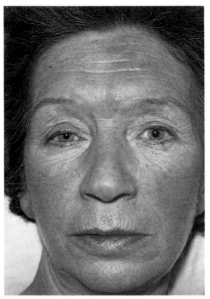

268

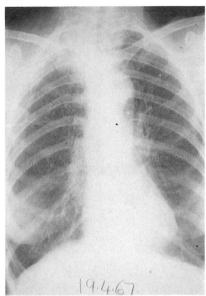

19.4.67.

269

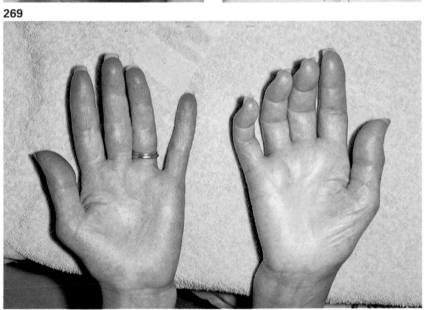

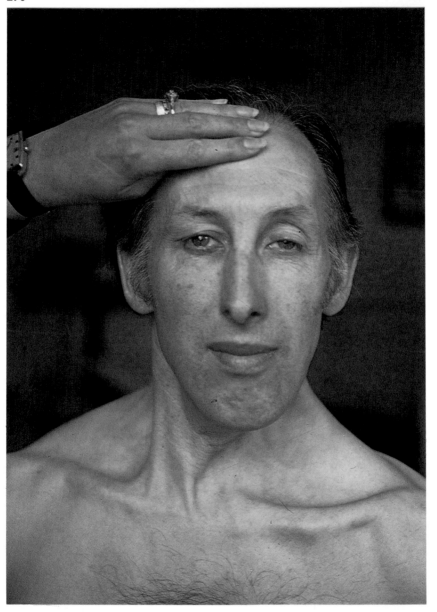

270 & 271 *Horner's syndrome with cranial nerve palsies* Left sided ptosis and no pupillary inequality (partial cervical sympathetic nerve lesion), the wasted left sternomastoid, particularly the clavicular head, and the wasted upper part left trapezius (supply: 11th cranial, spinal accessory nerve) and a left lower motor neurone hypoglossal nerve (12th cranial) palsy is apparent. The lesion is at the base of the skull.

This man presented with hoarseness (vagus palsy) and gradual involvement of the 12th and 11th nerves. At operation a neurofibroma on the 12th nerve was removed.

272 *Partial unilateral ptosis* Slight right sided ptosis is present without frontalis overaction and with small pupils. She had dysphagia. The lesion was in the brain stem.

271

272

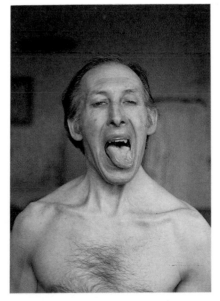

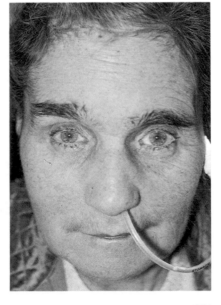

273 *Functional ptosis* This man has a complaint of a right sided drooping of the eyelid. The pupils are normal and there is frontalis overaction present on the opposite side to the ptosis: this should alert one to the possibility that it may be functional since it is impossible to simulate a ptosis without some elevation occurring of the opposite eyebrow.

274 & 275 *Third nerve palsy (encephalitis)* The ptosis is usually unilateral and may be partial or complete. The pupil is larger and fixed in a total palsy. The eye is deviated downwards (unopposed action of the superior oblique muscle – 4th nerve) and outwards (unopposed action of the lateral rectus – 6th nerve). There is a consequent inability to look inwards or upwards. Frontalis over reaction may be present.

Other causes are: mid brain lesions – vascular, encephalitic and of multiple sclerosis. In association with pain or headache the usual cause is an aneurysm of the posterior communicating cerebral artery. Non-painful causes include syphilis and diabetes.

273

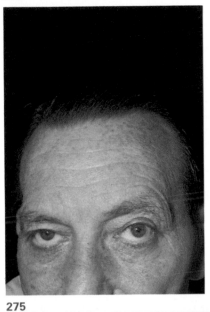

274

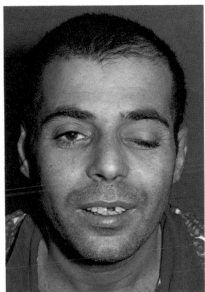

275

276 *Pseudo ptosis (contralateral lid retraction)* Thyrotoxic lid retraction with mild exophthalmos. The fallacy of supposing that the normal eye has a ptosis should be avoided. This patient presented complaining of a right sided drooping of the eyelid noticed by his wife when he looked over the top of the morning paper. In addition he had palpitations and a preference for cold weather. Always answer the question 'which is the abnormal side?'

277 *Tabes dorsalis* This slide shows a man demonstrating that he has an *abnormal range of movement*. This could be normal, e.g. if he is an acrobat, or he sits on the floor all day long and has very mobile hips. It could be due to ligamentous laxity, – the Peter Pan hypermobility syndrome or to a disorder of collagen rendering them lax as in pseudoxanthoma elasticum. He could be hypotonic, either due to a lower motor neurone paralysis, a cerebellar lesion or a posterior column lesion such as tabes dorsalis. He could have a disordered neuropathic joint with a painless abnormal range of movement. He also has *bilateral ptosis,* **251**.

276

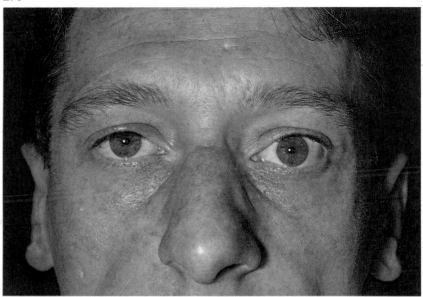

277

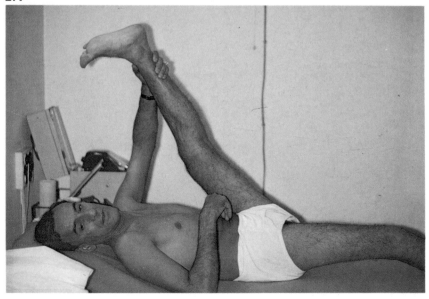

278–280 *Xanthelasmata* Lipid deposits under and round the eye associated with hyperlipoproteinaemia may occur without an underlying disorder.

These three patients cover the appearances of xanthelasmata which vary from an orange plaque to a fatty lump.

281 *Corneal arcus* Terminology based on the age of the patient is unsatisfactory. The arcus may be seen in association with hypercholesterolaemia, old age and occasionally in youth. It is related to lipid deposited in the corneal layers and may be a partial arc or a full circle. There is an association between age, the presence of an arcus and the chance of a myocardial infarction.

Lipid deposits. *Hypercholesterolaemia* may be secondary to (1) myxoedema, (2) nephrosis, (3) diabetes, (4) diet, (5) cholestasis, or be a primary disorder of lipid metabolism as may *hypertriglyceridaemia,* which also occurs in alcoholism, stress, diabetes. Tendon deposits are usually associated with hyperbetalipoproteinaemias, cutaneous xanthomas generally occur with associated additional hypertriglyceridaemias.

278

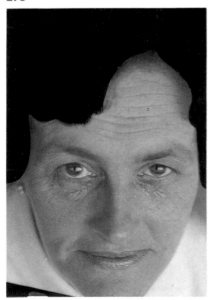

279

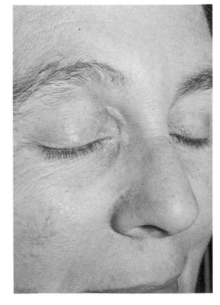

280

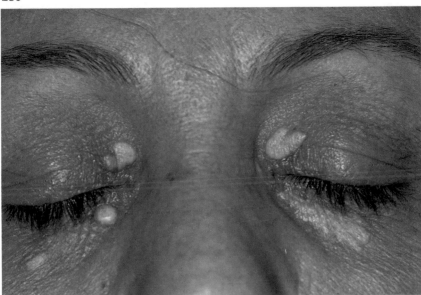

281

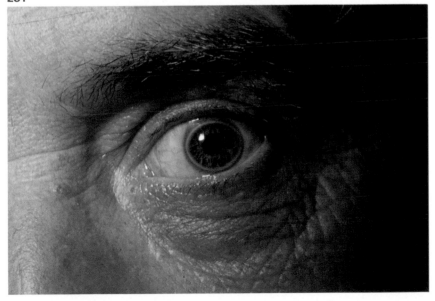

282 *Familial essential hypercholesterolaemia* There are deposits of tendon xanthomata seen in the hand of the patient with the arcus. These tendon xanthomata may be seen in association with cutaneous xanthomata. The tendons commonly affected are the Achilles and triceps insertion.

283 *Familial essential hypercholesterolaemia, type II[a]* A very marked arcus is seen. Always look for other related physical signs – xanthelasmata, tendon nodules. Serum cholesterol elevated (without other cause) and normal triglycerides are the diagnostic points.

284 *Asymptomatic tendon nodules* Unassociated with hyperlipoprotein-aemia from which they must be differentiated, or with any joint disorder. They are asymptomatic though they may antedate the appearance of a rheumatic condition by some years.

285 *Cutaneous xanthomata (xanthoma tuberosum)* Type III and familial dysbetalipoproteinaemia often seen in the buttocks, palms and elbows. Hypercholesterolaemia *and* raised triglycerides present.

282

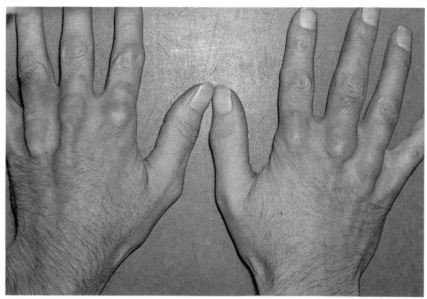

283

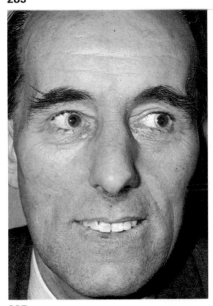

284

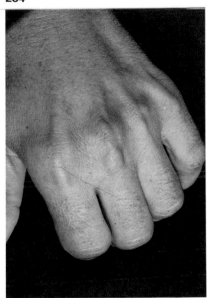

285

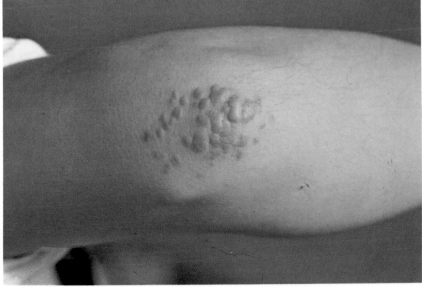

The appearance of the conjunctiva and sclera

Coloured sclera may be due to: (1) a thin sclera allowing choroidal pigment to show through – fragilitas ossium; (2) pigment deposited in the sclera either from an internal or external source, – silver, bilirubin, melanin; (3) increased vascularity.

286–288 *Fragilitas ossium* The father and son in **286** and **287** have blue sclerotics and repeated fractures. The Arab child in **288** shows a less marked colour change due to a thicker sclera.

286

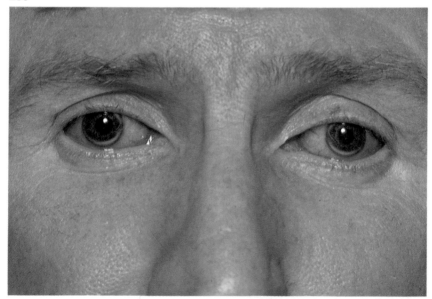

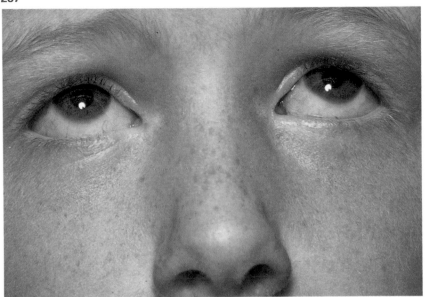

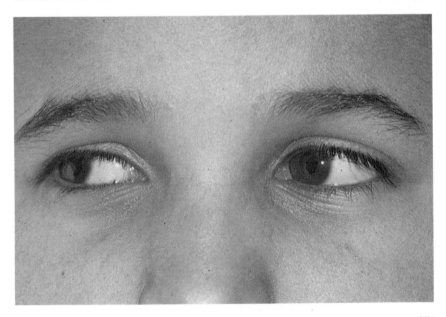

289 *Argyria (Bedouin Arab)* This eye has had silver nitrate eye drops placed in it for many years to combat the redness of the eye induced by climatic conditions. The silver has been deposited and pigments the sclera. Note that it affects both the conjunctival linings of the lower lid as well as the sclera itself. Circulating *bilirubin* will also stain the sclera and produce the classic jaundice tint from deepest yellow to palest lemon. The whiteness of the sclera will depend on the colour of the light reflected from it and therefore if the light has a yellow tinge minor degrees of yellowness of the conjunctivae will be missed.

290 & 291 *Acute conjunctivitis* Generalised injection and oedema (chemosis) affect the lower lid conjunctiva (**291**). Where the conjunctiva is least vascular a pale white ring is seen at the limbus (**290**).

292 *Acute glaucoma* The injection is around the limbus, the picture of uveitis, the redness here being less intense and more blue-red. Uveitis may be associated with systemic conditions, chronic infections like syphilis and tuberculosis, parasitic diseases such as toxoplasmosis, chronic granulomatous disease and the collagen diseases.

289

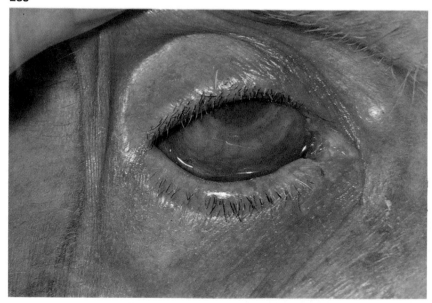

290

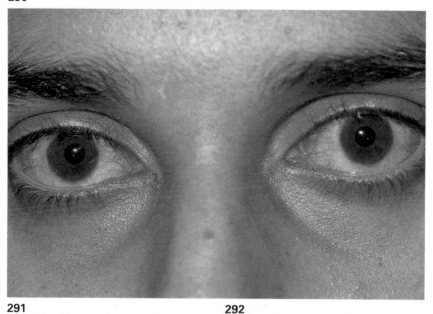

291

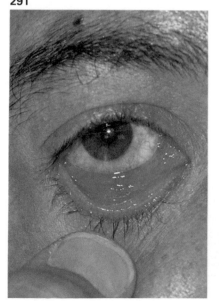

292

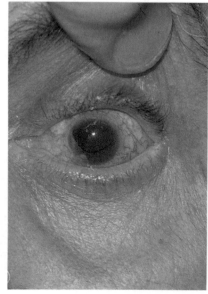

293 *Episcleritis* The redness is particularly marked at the inner limbic area, the dilated blood vessels being between the conjunctiva and the sclera. This is episcleritis, usually segmental, covering one or two quadrants, accentuated at the limbus and often associated with collagen disease. Note the petechiae in the lower lid conjunctiva in this patient who had disseminated lupus erythematosus.

294 & 295 *Pterygium* A benign leash of vessels and fibrous tissue which spreads across the eye and is only of importance when it passes across the cornea when it may interfere with vision. Figure **294** shows it before it has actually encroached on the cornea, and **295** has it encroaching on the cornea.

296 *Sub conjunctival haemorrhage* Note the blood, the posterior margin of which can be seen. This is a child with whooping cough, the rupture being precipitated by the straining, though it may occur spontaneously.

293

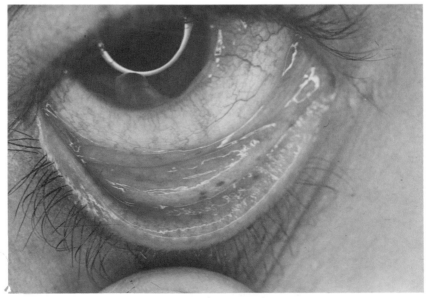

294

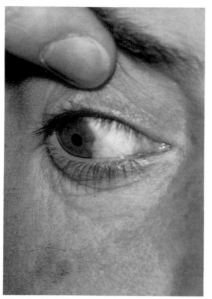

295

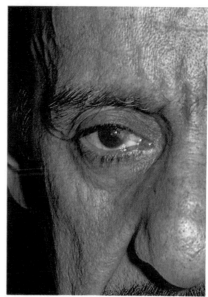

296

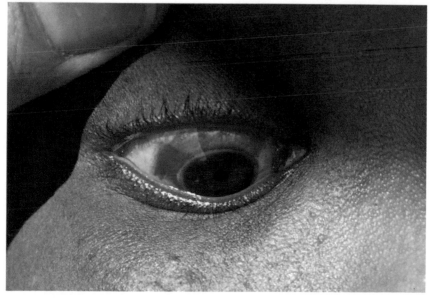

297 *Conjunctival haemorrhage* A small embolus has lodged in the conjunctival vessels and can be seen as a petechia. Abnormal bleeding is often seen in the conjunctivae where the blood vessels are unsupported.

298–299 *Kayser-Fleischer ring in Wilson's disease* The ring in a grey eye and a blue eye can be seen as a deposition of brown pigment at the margin of the corneal area. It may not be continuous as in these two cases but may only extend for part of the circle. The copper containing pigment is deposited on the posterior surface of the cornea, in Desçemet's membrane slightly away from the limbus so that a clear arc may exist between the ring and the corneoscleral junction. *(Samuel Alexander Kinnier Wilson, 1878–1936, described 1912; Bernard Kayser, 1869–1954, described 1902; Bruno Fleischer, German ophthalmologist, described 1903; Jean Desçemet, French anatomist, 1732–1810.)*

297

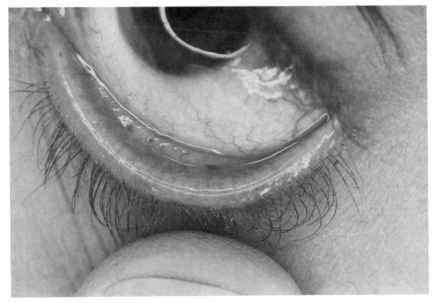

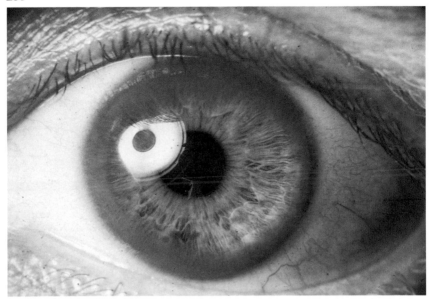

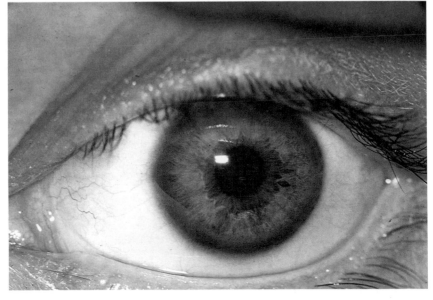

300 & 301 *Kayser-Fleischer ring in Wilson's disease* Compare these two eyes with **298** and **299** which show the rings in different degrees.

302 *Cataract* The classic cataract can be seen in this eye. Early cataracts may not be so obvious and will be seen with the ophthalmoscope when using the +12D lens for initial examination as central polar cataracts. The cataracts may be congenital or due to old age. They may be secondary to trauma, either physical or from ionising radiation, diabetes, hypocalcaemia or steroid therapy.

300

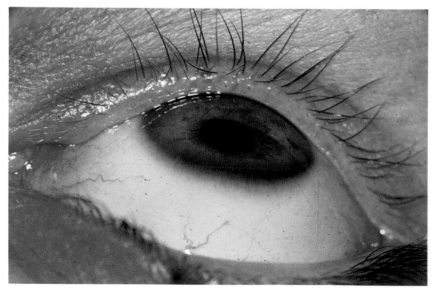

301

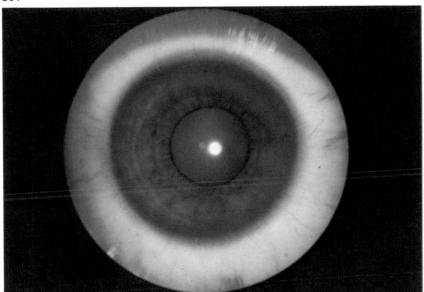

302

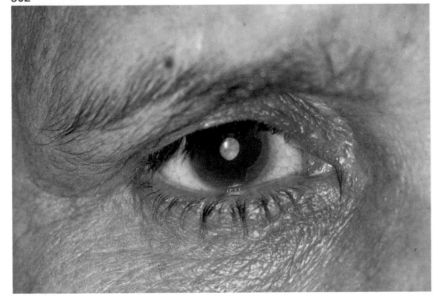

The pupils

303 *The large dilated pupil (atropine eye drops)* This may be unilateral or bilateral and may occur not only from eye drops but from contamination by the fingers with atropine-containing lotions, leading to blurred vision. It is also seen as a side effect of anti-hypertensive and cholinergic drugs.

Unilateral changes may be due to: (1) local causes – operations causing inflammation and adhesions, pupillary irregularity; (2) third nerve palsy – the pupillary dilation may recover early leaving the lateral deviation and the complete ptosis; (3) Horner's syndrome – in contrast to 2 the pupil is small, also associated with ptosis which is partial and with no external ocular palsy.

304 *Regular small pupils (treated chronic simple glaucoma)* Pinpoint small pupils, bilateral, should make one think of: (1) drug addiction, heroin; (2) glaucoma and instillation of pilocarpine; (3) Horner's syndrome, sympathetic palsy, but then they would not be so small; (4) pontine lesions; (5) sleep. Do not be misled into thinking that the small pupil of someone who is asleep is necessarily pathological.

303

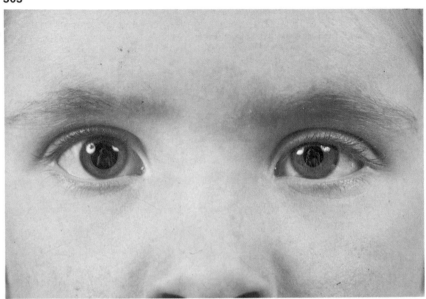

304

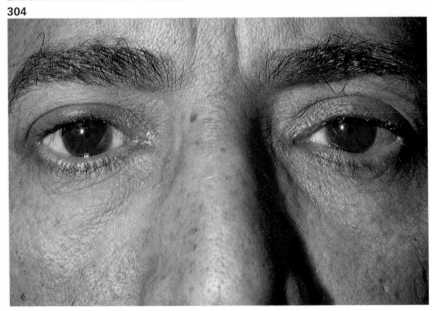

305 *Irregular unequal small pupils* The irregular pupil which is small and reacts poorly to light but briskly to convergence, slowly to mydriatics with depigmentation of the iris is the classic pupil of neuro-syphilis – the Argyll Robertson pupil.

306 *Argyll Robertson pupils* Here not only are the pupils irregular and small but the atrophy of the colour adjacent to the pupil can be seen. *(Douglas Moray Cooper Lamb Argyll Robertson, 1837–1909, described 1868, Edinburgh.)*

305

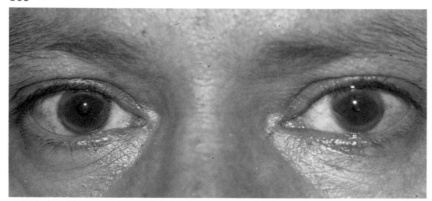

306

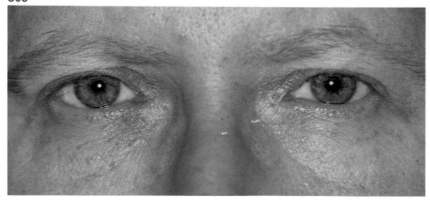

307 & 308 *Regular pupils reacting slowly to light* Holmes-Adie syndrome presenting as unequal but regular pupils. In the dark pupils are equal (**307**), after exposure to light the right pupil constricts, the left remains dilated (**308**). They both reacted to convergence. *(William John Adie, 1886–1935, described 1931; Gordon Holmes, described 1931.)*

307

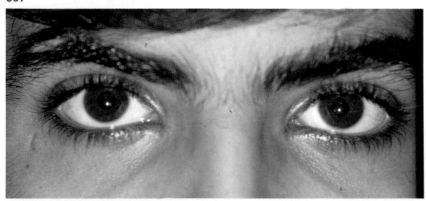

308

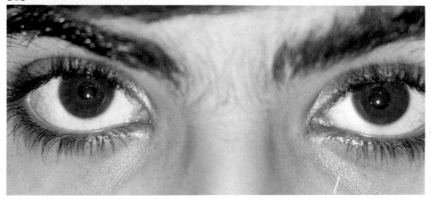

309

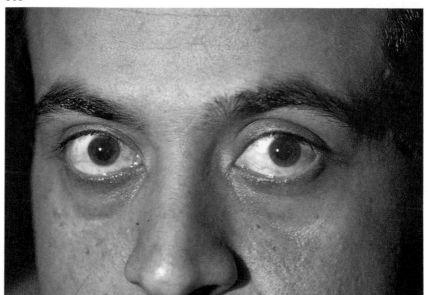

310

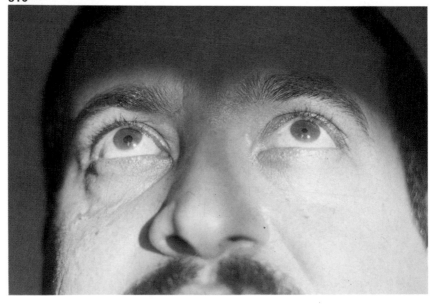

309 & 310 *Holmes-Adie syndrome, the myotonic pupil* In the dark the pupils are equal and dilated. In sunlight (**310**) the left pupil has constricted much more quickly than the right which comes down very slowly and once contracted will dilate again only slowly – the tonic pupil. It may be associated with absence of the tendon reflexes and is a benign condition which is important as a differential diagnosis from tabes dorsalis.

311 & 312 *Peripheral and broad iridectomy* The pupillary irregularity of the operation performed for increased ocular tension – glaucoma. A broad iridectomy (**312**) is performed in the eye affected by acute glaucoma particularly if iris atrophy occurs, the peripheral iridectomy is then performed prophylactically in the fallow eye to assist drainage (**311**). An iridectomy in only one of the pair suggests either old iritis and a broad iridectomy to sweep off the synechiae or a peripheral one as part of a cataract removal, in which case the eye will be aphakic.

311

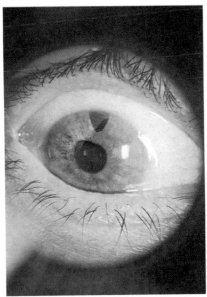

312

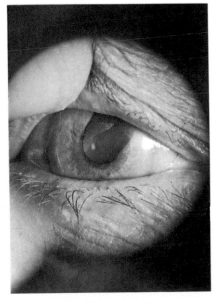

THE EARS

313 *Congenital absence or gross deformity of the pinna* This is usually associated with other changes in the first and second branchial arches when it may be associated with the Treacher-Collins syndrome, mandibulo-facial dystostosis. *(E. Treacher-Collins, described 1900, U.K.)*

314 *Accessory auricle* An interesting abnormality of no importance, sometimes requiring surgical excision for cosmetic reasons. They occur anteriorly to the tragus.

315 *Pre-auricular sinus* Remnant of the branchial cleft – may present as a swelling anterior to the tragus. Some dried exudate can be seen superior and anterior to the tragus (*arrow*) with surrounding brawny swelling.

316 *Pre-auricular sinus, uninfected* The dimple of the sinus can be seen at the arrow, superior and anterior to the tragus on the right of the picture. The track may extend deeply and may require extensive dissection. A thyroglossal duct track in the neck presents a similar surgical problem (see **545**).

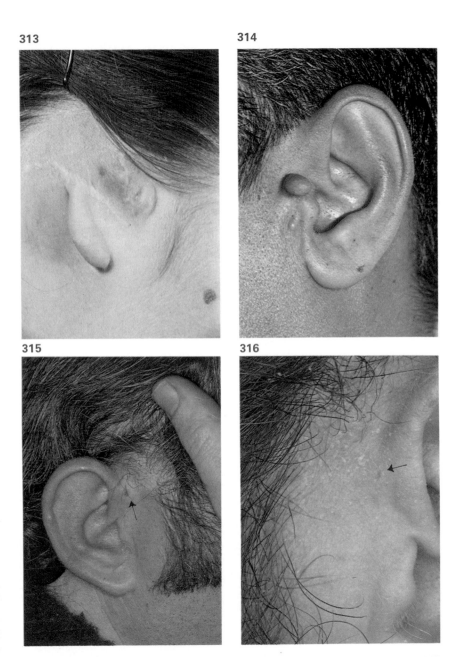

317 *Darwin's tubercle* A developmental remnant analogous to the tip of the mammalian ear, should not be confused with gouty tophi. The tubercle may be prominent as is seen here, or seen as a bump. (See **319**).

318 *Gouty tophus* The deposition of uric acid in the cartilage of the ear may be seen as small, white excrescences on the helix. They may be confused with Darwin's tubercle and should be looked for diligently. Here they are small and not obvious. *(Charles Darwin, 1809–1882.)*

319–321 *Gouty tophus* This one is easily seen and should be contrasted with the less prominent Darwin's tubercle (*arrowed*) of the ear. Needling and expression of the uric acid paste is diagnostic. It can be spread on a slide, as is seen, when the crystals may then be identified by their characteristic birefringence in polarised light.

317

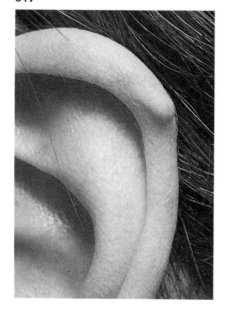

318

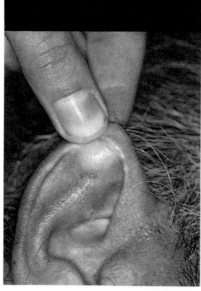

319

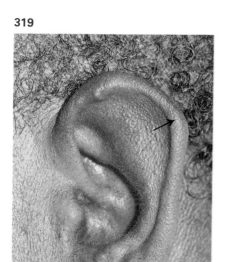

320

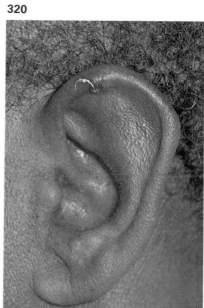

321

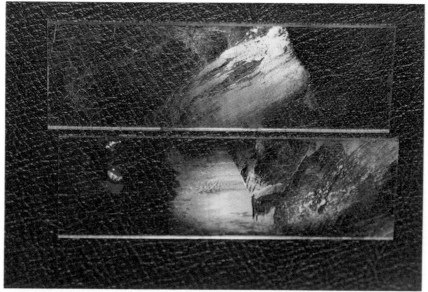

322 & 323 *The ear lobe* The lobe of the ear may be the site of keloid formation after ear piercing. It is also a common site for blood letting as a folk remedy for 'stroke', particularly in the Mediterranean area (**322**). This man developed a right sided hemiplegia and his daughter treated it by blood letting – opening the ear lobe with a razor blade.

324 *Haemangiomas of the pinna* Cavernous haemangiomas. Main importance is the differential diagnosis from lepromatous leprosy. Note the thickening of the ear, the change in colour and texture which also spreads on to the skin of the neck (*arrowed*). Compare this with the ear affected by lepromatous leprosy (**326**).

325 *Haemorrhagic telangiectasia* The pinna is a common site to see the dilated capillary loops in this condition.

326 *Lepromatous leprosy* Lepromatous leprosy produces a characteristic thickening of the ear. Note the change in skin texture. It is a common site for biopsy. It should not be confused with a capillary naevus which may affect the ear (**324**).

322

323

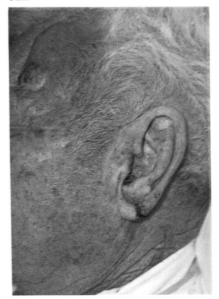

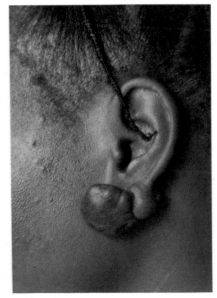

324

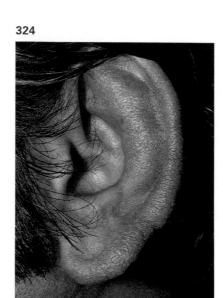

325

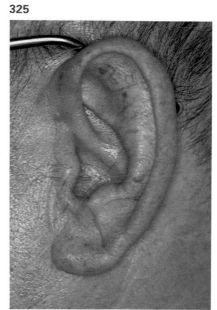

326

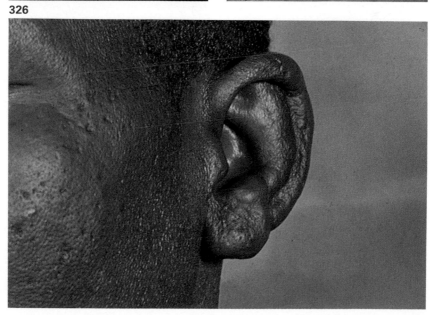

327 *Facial palsy and herpes* The Ramsay Hunt syndrome – a diagnostic point in the aetiology of the facial palsy. Note the vesicles in the external auditory meatus due to herpes zoster involving the geniculate ganglion of the seventh cranial nerve. The herpes will then affect the ear and pre-auricular region. *(James Ramsay Hunt, 1872–1937, described 1907.)*

328–331 *Ochronosis (alcaptonuria)* The ear has a grey cast from the pigmented cartilage showing through the skin. In this condition there is a deposition of the pigment in the cartilage – homogentisic acid – which may progress to calcification (**329**, and **330** lateral view, spine). This may be associated with premature osteo-arthrosis. The characteristic slate grey colour of the nodules can be seen through the skin (**331**). Nodules in the tendons may be due to: (1) rheumatoid arthritis; (2) gouty tophi; (3) xanthomata; (4) ochronosis.

327

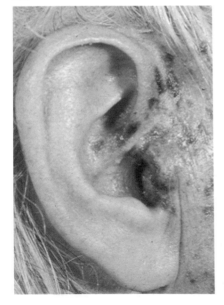

328

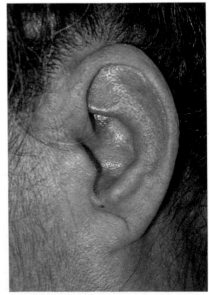

329

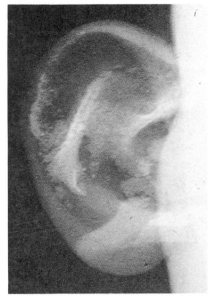

330

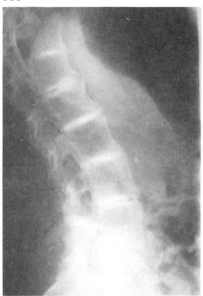

331

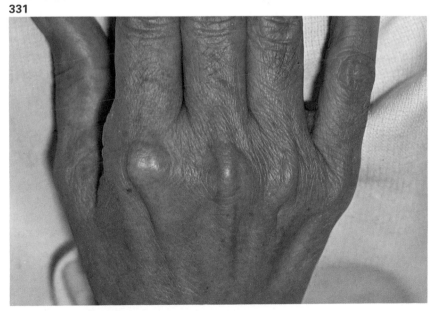

332 *Alcaptonuria* Alcaptonuria – an inborn error of metabolism – is the predecessor of ochronosis, the deposition of the oxidised black/brown pigment of homogentisic acid – which binds irreversibly with collagen and alters its physical properties and leads to degenerate changes. The urine oxidises on exposure to air: these specimens being passed through a 24 hour period and demonstrating the darkening with standing – the oldest is on the left.

Urine colour changes

Dilute urine – *white*

Concentrated urine – *yellow/orange*

Bile in the urine – *yellow/orange*

Haemoglobinuria – *red*

Beetroot – *red/pink*

Alcaptonuria – *yellow/grey on standing*

Porphyria – *darkened on standing, dark red (fluorescent, **333**)*

Phenolthalein in alkaline urine – *red*

Melanuria – *black*

Methaemoglobinuria – *black*

Methylene blue – *green/blue*

333 *Porphyria* The urine darkens on standing (port wine) and fluoresces in ultra-violet light. On the left a control and patient's urine and on the right patient's stool and control.

332

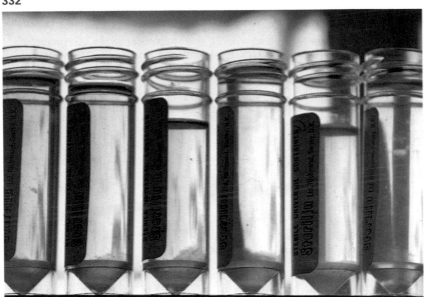

333

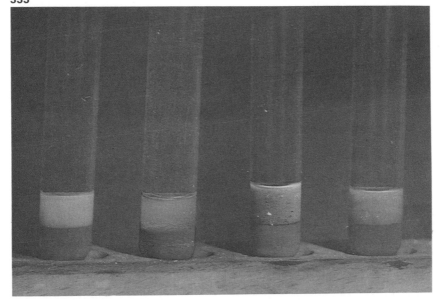

334 *Achondroplasia* The skull is of approximately normal size though large in contrast to the body. The bridge of the nose is depressed and the nostrils tend to point outwards. A characteristic skull shape occurs in: microcephaly, small; hydrocephalus, big; rickets, thickened osteoid seams at suture – 'hot cross bun'; osteitis deformans, Paget's (**132, 221**); haemoglobinopathy, thickened bone (**34, 136**); acromegaly, overgrowth (**117**).

335 *Acute ethmoiditis* Acute sinusitis can produce swelling and nasal deformity. This man had acute ethmoiditis. Note the widening of the bridge of the nose and oedema.

336 *Sarcoidosis* She has lupus pernio of the nose, bone cysts on the fingers, and blindness secondary to iritis. All manifestations of sarcoidosis.

334

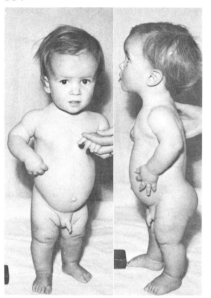

335

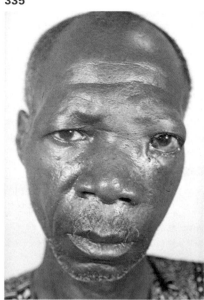

336

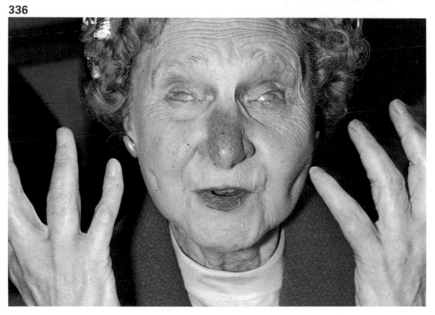

THE MOUTH

The entrance to the gut. This is an area, like the hand, where information and pathological changes are concentrated.

337 *Osler-Weber-Rendu disease (congenital haemorrhagic telangiectasia)* Male, 60-years-old, repeatedly investigated for bleeding including laparotomy. Finally had an operation and then suffered from malabsorption. His luxuriant moustache was eventually removed and the diagnosis was only then made when the telangiectases were seen around the mouth. *(Sir William Osler, 1849–1919, described 1907; Frederick Parkes Weber, 1863–1962, described 1904; Henri Jules Louis Marie Rendu, 1844–1902, described 1896.)*

338 *Peutz-Jeghers syndrome* Melanin pigmentation as spots around the lips and mouth. Associated with intestinal polyps. *(J L A Peutz, Germany, described 1921; Harold Jeghers, described 1949.)*

339 *Peutz-Jeghers syndrome* These spots appear like freckles, and extend onto the lips and buccal mucosa (**340**).

337

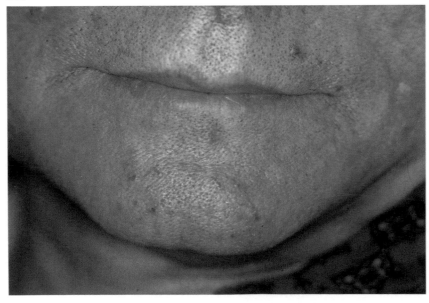

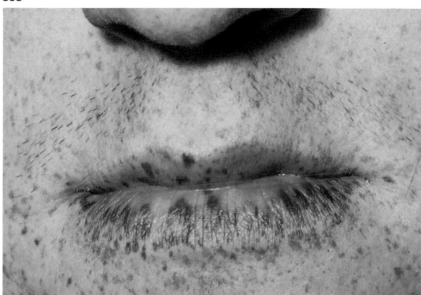

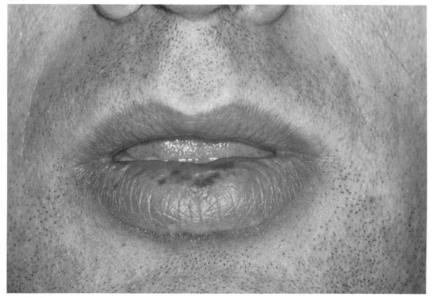

340 *Peutz-Jeghers syndrome* The freckle-like spots on the buccal mucosa. They may also be seen on the hands and may be sparse or profuse.

341 *Central cyanosis (mild)* Colour changes in the blood are easily seen in the vermilion border of the lip – the plethora of polycythaemia must not be confused with cosmetics, the chewing of coloured substances such as betel which stain the lip and the sucking of lollipops by children which can render the lip any colour.

Cyanosis due to decreased oxygen saturation of haemoglobin (less than 85%) may be noted in the extremities but differentiation into central cyanosis can only be achieved by examination of the colour of the lips which are usually warm, and better still the tongue. *Central cyanosis* may be due to: (1) lung disease with defective oxygenation; (2) congenital shunts and mixing of arterial and venous blood; (3) increased red cell populations, excess reduced red cells. *Peripheral cyanosis* – blue ears and blue fingers are so often due to peripheral vasoconstriction from cold, consequent sluggish circulation and desaturation of the blood.

This young woman has central cyanosis secondary to primary pulmonary hypertension.

340

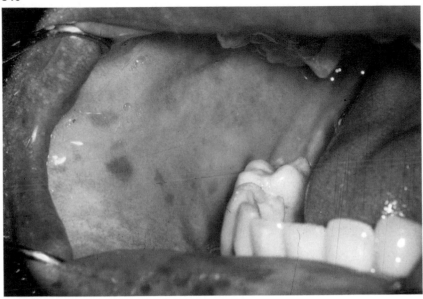

341

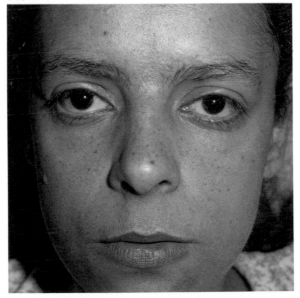

342 & 343 *Methaemoglobinaemia* The tongue has a blue tint. The patient suffers from methaemoglobinaemia due to the ingestion of phenacetin. One week later when the methaemoglobinaemia had cleared the tongue had returned to a normal colour and the haemoglobin had reverted to normal. This is an example of toxic acquired methaemoglobinaemia, usually secondary to the ingestion of aromatic amino or nitro compounds and of aniline dyes in laundry marks and waxed crayons. It will produce symptoms of anoxia. 1.2–2g/100ml of methaemoglobin in the blood will produce visible cyanosis compared with 5g of deoxygenated haemoglobin required to produce true cyanosis.

344 *Angular stomatitis* There is a cracking at the angle of the mouth which may become indolent and infected. This is commonly seen in: (1) malnutrition; (2) vitamin B and folate deficiency; (3) habitual licking of the lips in children; (4) the older patient whose poorly fitting teeth, or lack thereof, allows overclosure and apposition of the corners of the mouth which become soggy.

All of these may become secondarily infected with monilia.

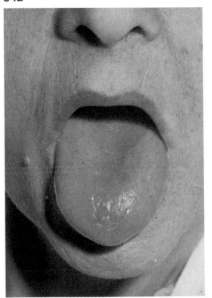

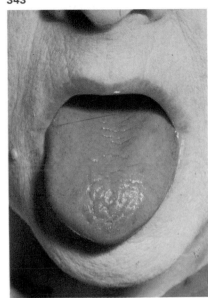

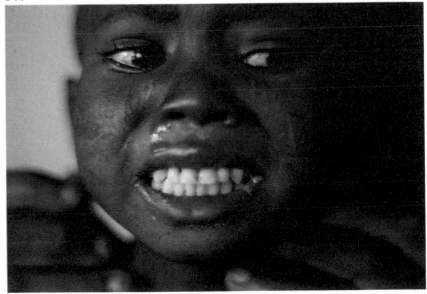

345 *Angular stomatitis* Secondary to habitual licking of the lips with the tongue. Super infection with monilia has occurred.

346 *The cold sore (herpes febrialis or herpes simplex)* This common eruption seen on the lip is due to activation of the herpes virus and presents as a vesicle on a red base which ruptures and crusts. The time course is about seven days from start to finish. It is commonly associated with febrile conditions and classically is seen in pneumonia. Primary herpetic infection may be associated with moderate regional glandular enlargement. The time interval in these two views was four days.

345

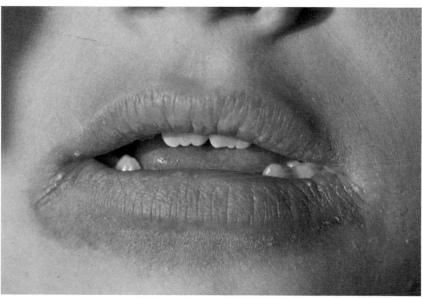

346

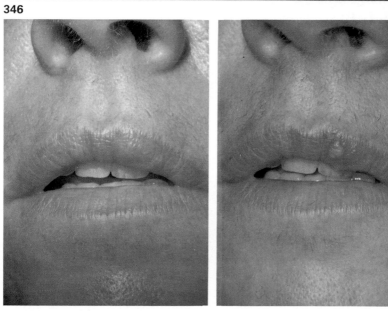

347 *Primary syphilitic chancre of the lip* Ulcers on the lip may be traumatic, infective or malignant (basal cell carcinoma) in origin.

348 *Congenital syphilis* Peri-oral patches at the margins of the mouth heal and lead to scarring known as *rhagades*. The angular stomatitis of malnutrition does not scar.

347

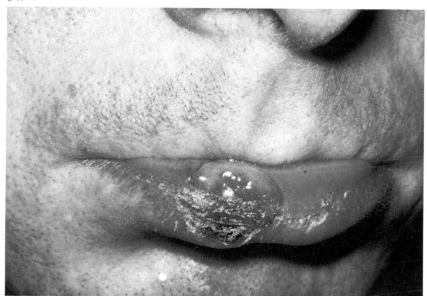

348

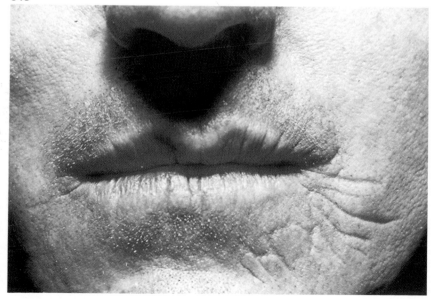

349 *Angio-neurotic oedema of the lip* This is a common site for allergic swellings to take place which may be secondary to drugs, to insect stings or other allergies. A similar appearance may occur following trauma.

350 *Acromegaly* Soft tissue overgrowth produces a big fleshy lower lip which is further thrown into prominence by the prognathic jaw – compare the lip with the patient's driving licence photograph taken two years earlier (**116**).

351 *Mumps (unilateral parotid swelling)* A short history suggests an inflammatory cause (viral – mumps; bacterial – parotitis). An intermittent swelling suggests a calculus in the duct, and a long standing swelling suggests a tumour.

352 *Mumps* Examine the parotid duct orifice – in mumps it is often red and inflamed. In the debilitated patient with bacterial parotitis a drop of pus may be seen.

349

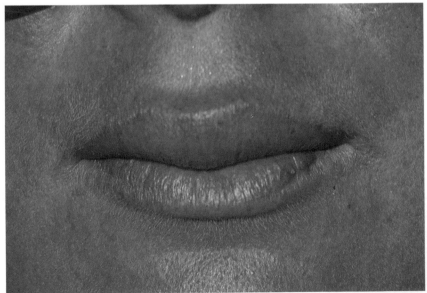

350

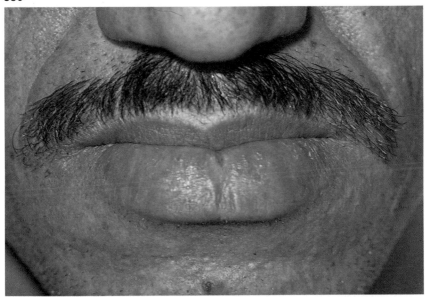

351

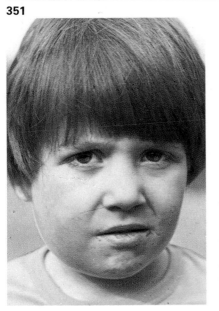

352

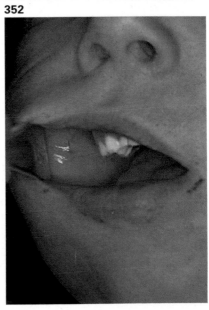

353 *Salivary duct calculus* Unilateral intermittent parotid swelling due to a salivary calculus. The swelling is related to retained saliva and to intermittent inflammation.

354 *Sub-mandibular salivary gland enlargement* Unilateral swelling of a salivary gland of long standing suggests a tumour.

355 *Bilateral parotid gland involvement (sarcoidosis)* This woman had enlargement of long duration due to sarcoidosis.

356 *Sarcoidosis* Parotid enlargement. Dry tongue and keratoconjunctivitis 'sicca' of Sjögren's syndrome. Long standing bilateral gland enlargement suggests sarcoidosis or infiltration with a lymphoma.

353

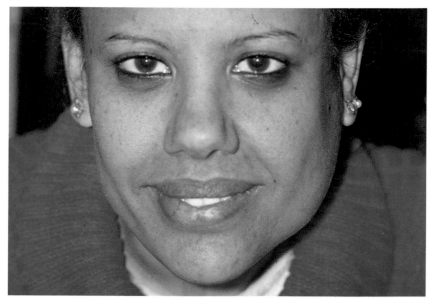

354

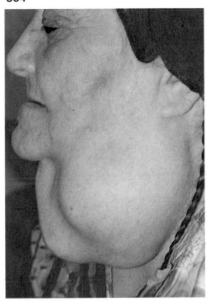

355

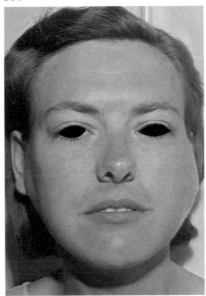

356

The gums

Infection: caused by poor dental hygiene. *Recession:* also a consequence of poor dental hygiene. *Hypertrophy:* a result of drugs (e.g. phenytoin). *Bleeding:* infection, scurvy, blood dyscrasia. *Poisoning:* heavy metals (lead produces brownish black discoloration at the gum margin).

357 *Gum recession* With age and poor dental hygiene the gum may recede and be helped by the recurrent episodes of infection between gum and tooth. Here the gum has receded and the exposed dentine is stained by nicotine.

358 *Periodontal inflammation (acromegaly)* May complain of pain, burning or bleeding – sometimes due to specific Vincent's infection. Initially red inflamed line seen around the tooth with small amounts of pus exuding between gum and tooth.

359 *Asymmetric gum recession (arrow)* Usually due to faulty teeth cleaning technique and the abrasive effect of the initial toothbrush stroke. It is one way of determining the dominant hand! A right handed brusher pulls the brush horizontally vigorously across the teeth and exerts most pull pressure at the beginning of the stroke on the left hand side. A left hander will produce right sided recession.

357

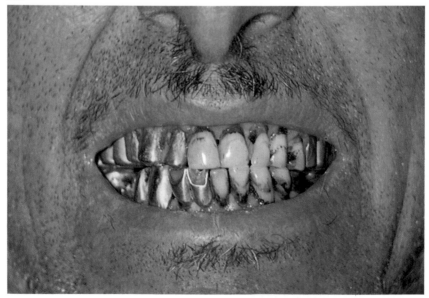

358

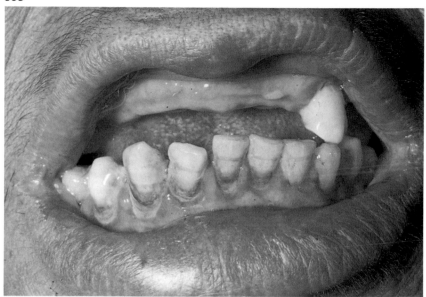

359

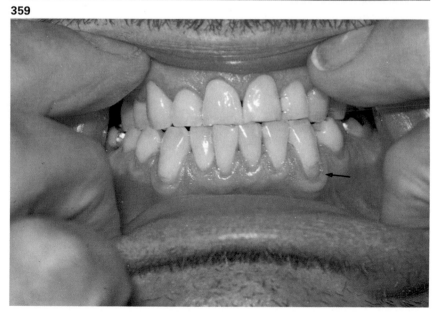

360 *Gum recession* Complete recession and re-absorption of the bone allows the teeth to fall. Note the exposed root and the re-absorption of the bone in a patient with a rare hereditary condition of the Papillon Lefeuvre syndrome where the early re-absorption and loss of the teeth is associated with hyperkeratosis of the palms and soles.

361 *Gum hypertrophy* Gum hypertrophy in a patient on anticonvulsant therapy with phenytoin.

362 *Bleeding gums* This is to be seen in (1) pyorrhoea, (2) scurvy, (3) bleeding diathesis. This patient with leukaemia also has extensive herpes.

360

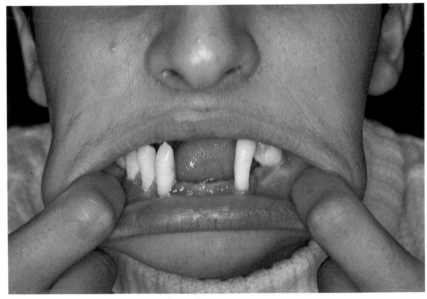

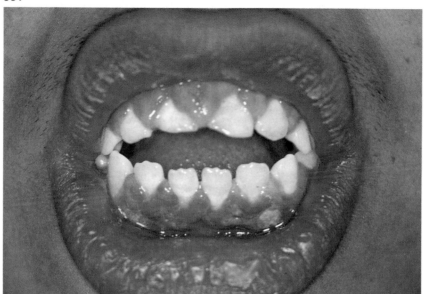

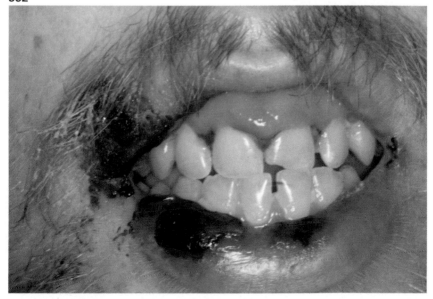

Teeth deformity is produced by (1) grinding – either in eating hard foods or deliberately for cosmetic reasons; (2) infection during development.

363–365 *Discoloured teeth (fluorosis)* There is discoloration of the enamel of the teeth with slight pitting. The patient came from an area where there was a high quantity of fluoride in the water. The fluoride is incorporated into the enamel and stains in high concentration, though increasing resistance to caries. Examination of the teeth is seldom a major help in diagnosis apart from the classic dental signs of syphilis. Insight into the patient may be gained by the sight of neglected teeth, nicotine staining and carious stumps.

Note: (1) Nicotine discoloration can be scraped off. (2) The ingestion of tetracycline whilst the enamel is being laid down produces a characteristic yellow discoloration (**364**). (3) Fluorosis produces a brown discoloration of the enamel (**363**). (4) Measles produces a changed density of enamel and may mark that enamel which was being made at the time of infection. Analogous to Beau's lines in the nails (**365**).

363

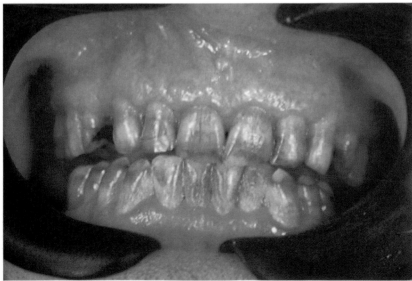

364

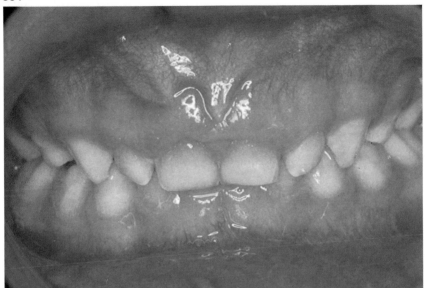

365

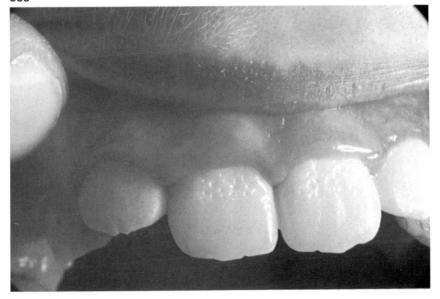

366

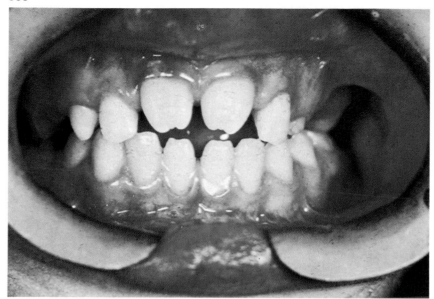

367

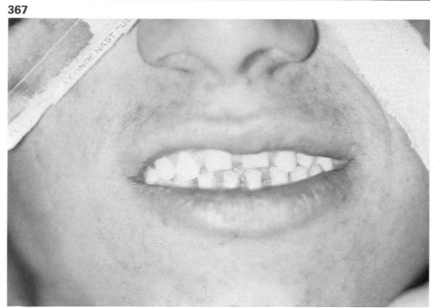

366 *Hutchinson's teeth (syphilis)* Infection with the spirochaete at the time of development of the permanent dentition results in deformity of the teeth as the infection interferes with the nutrition and causes suppression of the middle of the three denticles from which the tooth develops. The lateral denticles expand to fill the gap but do not succeed completely. Therefore the incisors are smaller, are widely spaced (if the maxilla is not shrunken), and have rounded or converging sides in screwdriver-like manner. The thinner enamel means that they wear easily and therefore become notched. It is usually the upper central and lateral and lower central and lateral incisors that are affected.

367 *Hutchinson's teeth* The lower incisors are straight sided and small: in consequence widely spaced in a normal sized jaw. The upper central incisors have a screwdriver tip shape; they appear widely spread. If the maxilla is hypoplastic due to congenital infections then the spacing will appear normal. Contrast this with acromegaly (**122**) where the teeth are of normal size but because of overgrowth of the lower jaw became widely spaced. This young girl has the left eye bandaged because of corneal grafting performed for interstitial keratitis. She was not deaf.

Hutchinson's triad in congenital syphilis: teeth; interstitial keratitis; deafness.

368

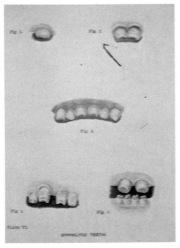

368 *Hutchinson's teeth* The original illustration of Hutchinson's teeth showing the different appearances depending on the state of wear of the teeth. *(Syphilis, J Hutchinson, 1887.)*

(Sir Jonathan Hutchinson, surgeon, London Hospital, 1828–1913, described 1858.)

The inside of the mouth may be the site of ulcers, emboli, inflammation, enanthemata or may show the colour changes of anaemia, cyanosis or pigmentation.

369 *Addison's disease* Classical brown pigmentation in Addison's disease occurs on the oral mucosa. It must be differentiated from the freckle pigmentation of Peutz-Jeghers disease (**338**). The increased pigmentation is due to stimulation of the melanocytes by raised levels of ß melanocyte stimulating hormone (ßMSH) which accompanies the raised ACTH level secondary to the low cortisol. ßMSH has amino acids in common with ACTH and so very high levels of ACTH produced by daily injection of synthetic ACTH (tetracosactrin) may produce an increase in pigmentation. Vitiligo (**55**) occurs in 15% of patients with Addison's disease.

370 *Pigmentation of the buccal mucosa* A woman with a very high level of ACTH secondary to parental therapy for asthma with synthetic ACTH. One should be careful since patches of pigment may be seen in the inner borders of the mouth which are in fact racial in origin.

371 *Palatal pigmentation* This man, a brown skinned Arab, was perfectly well and had pigmentation of the palate. Compare this with the pigmentation in Addison's disease (**369**). Local pigmentation of oral mucosa may often be an incidental finding.

The *differential diagnosis* of pigmentation includes: (1) Local – Peutz-Jeghers syndrome; Addison's disease. (2) Generalised – gastrointestinal disease (regional ileitis, ulcerative colitis, cirrhosis); neurofibromata; chronic debilitating disease (malignancy, TB, malabsorption malnutrition); endocrine disorders (Cushing's syndrome, thyrotoxicosis).

369

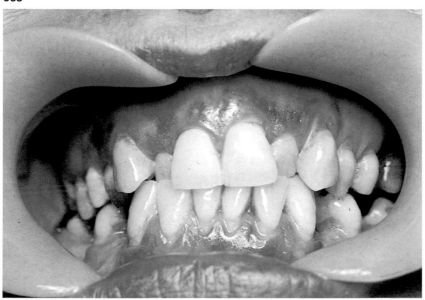

370

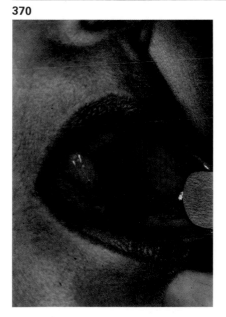

371

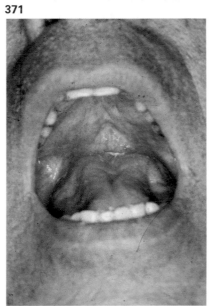

372 *Emboli of the hard palate* A case of septicaemia. Petechiae all look the same but the mouth is a characteristic site.

373 & 374 *Moniliasis (oral thrush)* An infection with moniliasis may occur in the debilitated, in babies and in those on broad spectrum antibiotics. It may be a continuous white membrane which brushes off and leaves a red base which does not bleed – or it may be punctate (**374**).

372

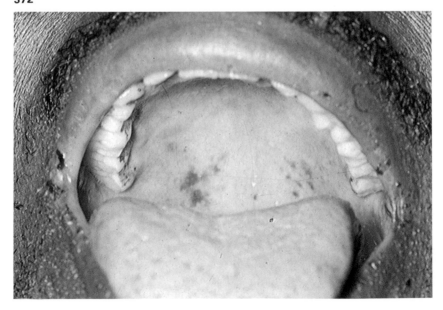

373

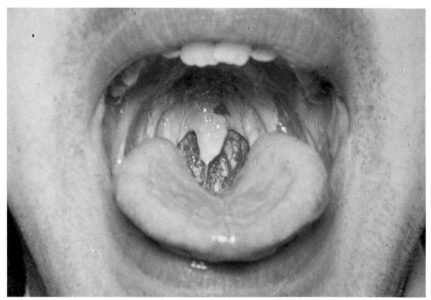

374

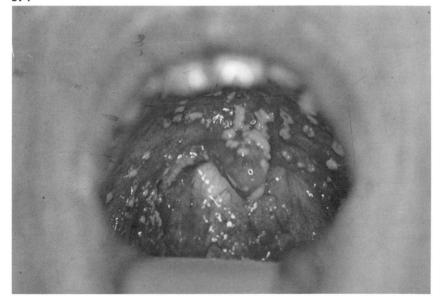

375 & 376 *Oral thrush* Debilitated Indian woman on steroids: diagnosis – systemic lupus erythematosus.

377 *Leukoplakia of the buccal mucosa* It may be secondary to poorly fitting dentures and is often seen opposite to an incompletely erupted wisdom tooth which is biting on the mucosa. Classically it is seen in those who take spices, smoke much or have syphilis. These white patches cannot be wiped off and biopsy should be performed since the condition is pre-malignant, as well as being a pointer to the presence of syphilis.

375

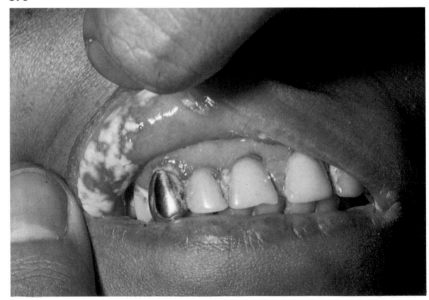

376

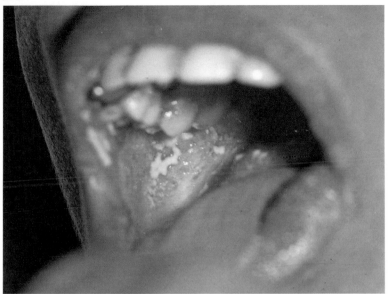

377

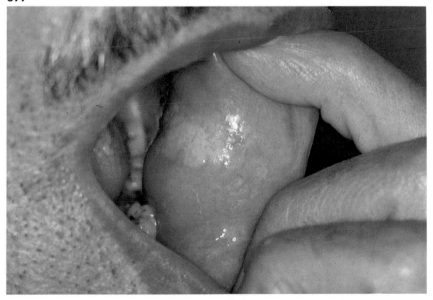

Common viral diseases have manifestations in the mouth. They may precede the main diagnostic eruption as in measles, or co-exist with it as in chicken pox.

378 *Koplik's spots* The enanthem of measles precedes the main rash by several days. Usually seen opposite the molars or on the buccal surface of the lips and cheeks. The spots resemble a grain of salt on the pink mucosa with a narrow halo of more intense red around them.

379 *Chicken pox* The spots are not confined to the skin and occur in the tongue and buccal mucosa at the same time as the main rash.

380–382 *Aphthous ulcers* Small ulcers, 1–4mm in diameter may occur on healthy persons as a recurrent, painful, self-limiting problem lasting five to six days, aetiology unknown. Behçet's disease (**382**) may show similar appearances in the mouth, but on occasion are larger and lead to scarring. Genital ulcers are also present as well as more generalised neurological or cardiovascular disease. An aphthous-like ulcer may occur on the pharynx in infectious mononucleosis (**385**). *(Halushi Behçet, 1889–1948, described 1937.)*

378

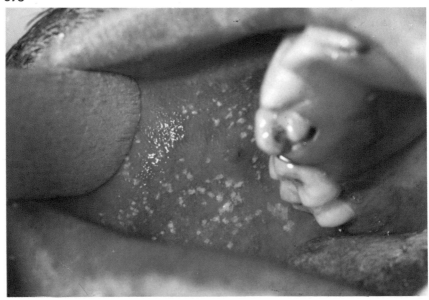

379

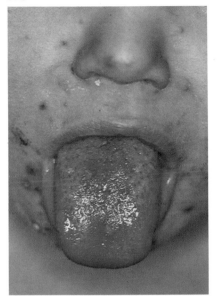

380

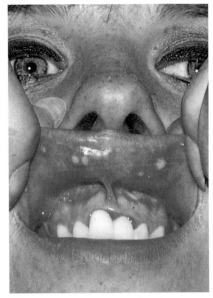

381

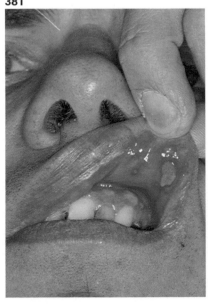

382

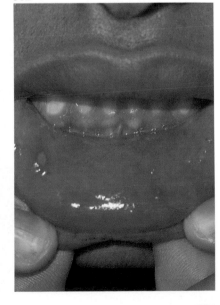

383 *Acute tonsillitis*

384 *Acute pharyngitis* The red, raw pharynx, either due to chronic irritation, smoking, or acute viral or bacterial infection.

385 *Infectious mononucleosis* A sore throat with petechiae and small ulcers may be seen in infectious mononucleosis.

386 *Ampicillin rash, infectious mononucleosis* The pharyngitis of mono-nucleosis may be inadvertently treated with ampicillin and show no improvement. The appearance of the irritating macular/papular rash due to ampicillin hypersensitivity suggests the diagnosis as sensitivity occurs more frequently in association with infectious mononucleosis.

383

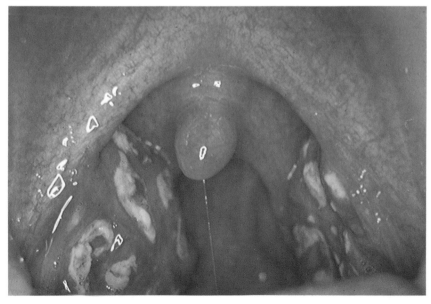

384

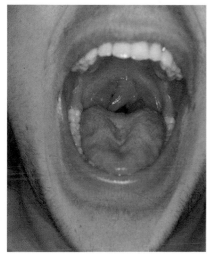

385

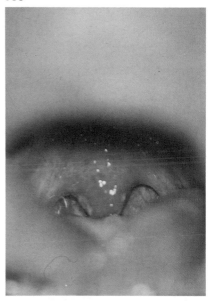

386

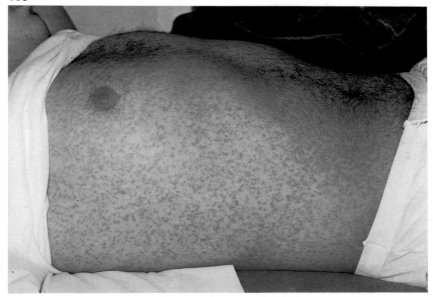

387 *Tonsillar diphtheria* In sore throats *never* forget this possibility – keep a high index of suspicion.

'Membrane is confined to the tonsils where absorption of toxin is moderate. It starts as a small patch on one tonsil and usually spreads to involve both. The membrane is ivory-white or greyish-yellow in colour. The edge is wrinkled but sharply demarcated and bordered by a narrow band of inflammation.

The child is listless and off-colour but may not complain of a sore throat and the cause of the illness may be overlooked. Pyrexia is slight or absent.' *(Emond. 'A Colour Atlas of Infectious Diseases' 1974.)*

388 & 389 *Cancrum oris* A breakdown in mucosal integrity with infection usually due to a fusiform bacillus with consequent gangrene and sloughing. It is common in Africa, often related to exanthemata of small children who are already on the borderlines of malnutrition. They are ill and have dehydrated mouths and the condition progresses rapidly through the stage of early swelling (**388**) to gangrene (**389**), sloughing (**390, 391**), contracture and healing (**392**). In **388** the necrotic tissue extends on the inside of the mouth and swelling alone is seen at this stage. The corner of the child's mouth has been torn by the insertion of the gag at the time of a febrile convulsion. In **389** (a different case) the necrosis has extended through the cheek and the dead tissue is about to slough.

387

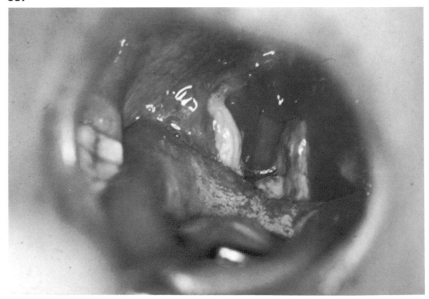

388

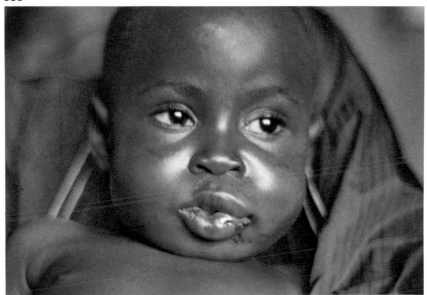

389

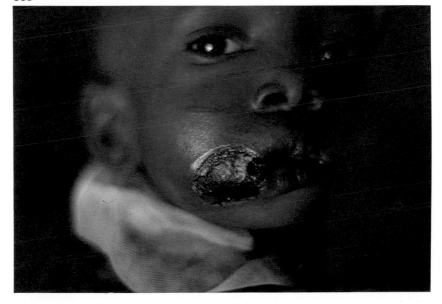

390 *Cancrum oris* Sloughing has taken place and will leave a vast defect in the cheek. The child himself remains relatively well.

391 *Cancrum oris* A small defect has sloughed, leaving a clean hole.

392 *Cancrum oris* The stage of healing and contraction. This had occurred during a recent febrile illness, probably smallpox.

393 *Ranula* This is a mucocoele of the floor of the mouth and may cause some confusion in diagnosis to the physician. The basic pathology is that of a retention cyst. The treatment is by excision.

390

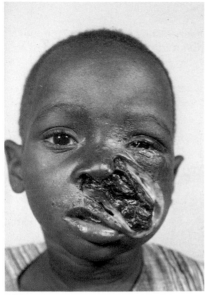

391

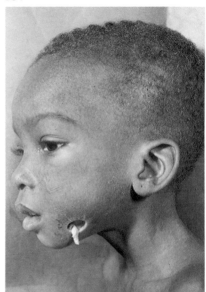

392

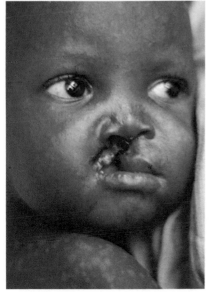

393

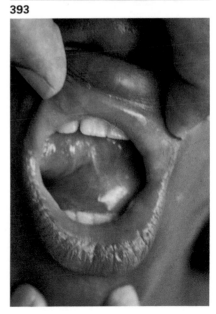

213

THE TONGUE

394 *Normal tongue* Clean, moist, with normal papillae.

395 *A normal coated tongue* Nicotine staining. The coating of the tongue may be of little significance, being related to mouth breathing, cigarette smoking or unknown factors.

396 *Geographical tongue* This is due to losses of papillae which regrow again and appear to migrate, hence the term geographical tongue, erythema migrans.

397 *Scrotal or fissured tongue* Another normal variant.

398 *Mongolism (Down's syndrome)* A high incidence of transverse fissuring of the tongue.

399 *Atrophy of papillae* May be associated with disease. The tongue is clean and smooth but the normal papillae are lost. Associated with pernicious anaemia, malabsorption or antibiotic therapy.

394

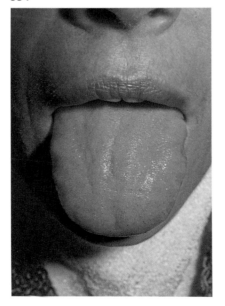

395

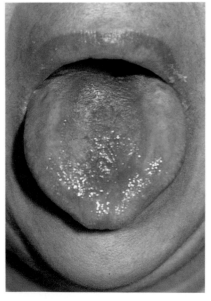

396

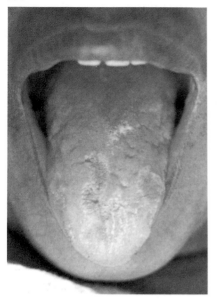

397

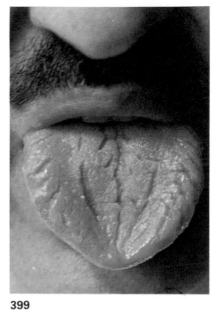

398

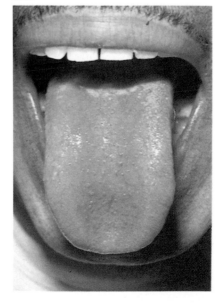

399

400 *Glossitis, vitamin B deficiency* A bright red sore tongue.

401 *The hairy tongue* Minor version – pigment usually being due to overgrowth with aspergillus niger, also occurs directly related to smoking.

402 *Hairy tongue* More marked.

403 *Dehydration* The dry tongue may reflect mouth breathing or inadequate oral toilet as well as systemic dehydration and diminished salivary flow. The white patches on the lateral borders are due to monilia.

404 *The sicca syndrome* A bone-dry tongue – xerostomia. This is one component of the syndrome described by Sjögren of dry eyes, dry tongue, and rheumatoid arthritis. It may occur in association with other autoimmune diseases and, as in this patient, in sarcoidosis. *(Henrik Samuel Conrad Sjögren, born 1899, described 1933.)*

405 *Leukoplakia of the tongue* Stratified squamous epithelium if chronically irritated by chemical (spices), thermal (smoking), infective (syphilis), or mechanical (dental irritation) agents responds by thickening and hyperkeratinisation with the formation of white patches – leukoplakia. Transition into squamous cell carcinoma may occur and biopsy is essential.

400

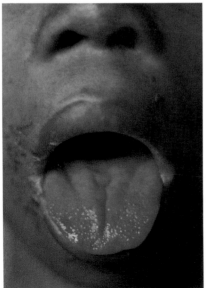

401

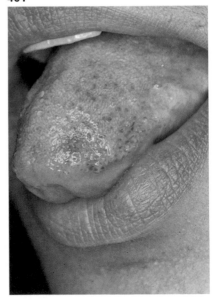

402

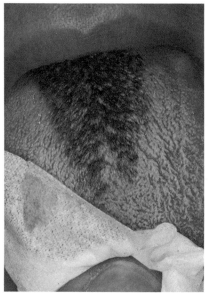

403

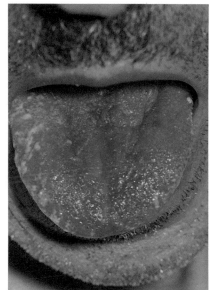

404

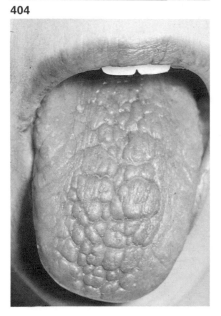

405

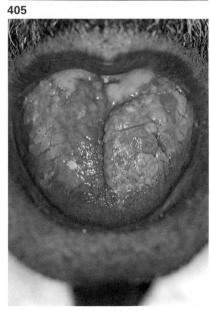

406 *Tongue tie* The fraenum is attached near to the end of the tongue. It is of no significance.

407 *Macro glossia (acromegaly)* A big tongue may be seen in acromegaly, amyloidosis and cretinism.

408 *The deviated tongue* Deviation occurs *towards* the weak side secondary to the unopposed action of the normal side. It is found in hypoglossal palsy or with an upper motor neurone lesion of that side. Bilateral upper motor neurone lesions produce an apparently small spastic tongue.

409 & 410 *Hypoglossal nerve palsy* Figure **408** shows a mild palsy and **409** and **410** a gross one. In **409** note the wasting where the longitudinal folds are exaggerated. Protrusion (**410**) by the normal genioglossus pushes the tongue to the affected side.

Unilateral lower motor neurone lesions produced by: (1) trauma (gunshot wounds); (2) brain stem lesions (syringobulbia, tumours); (3) tumours or glands at the base of the skull.

406

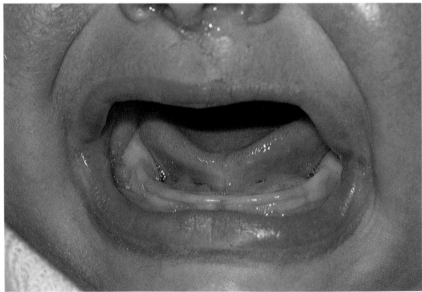

407

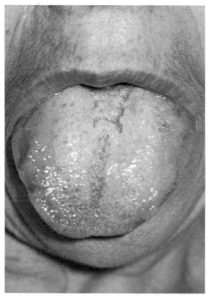

408

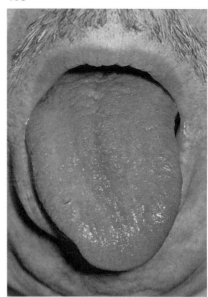

409

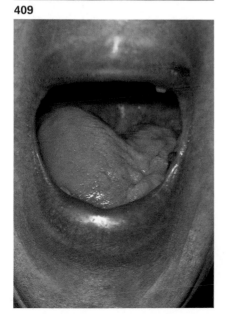

410

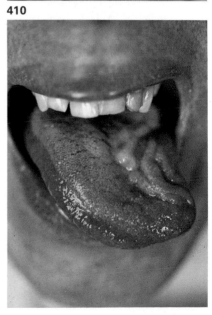

The Hands

The hand is like a blackboard on which the physical signs of disease affecting many systems may be seen, as well as social and occupational clues about the patient.

Anatomy

So much can be deduced by remembering a few basic neuroanatomical facts.

    (1) THENAR muscles: supplied by the MEDIAN nerve.
    (2) HYPOTHENAR muscles: supplied by the ULNAR nerve.
    (3) The radial nerve DOES NOT supply muscles in the hand.

The ULNAR nerve enters the hand and supplies the hypothenar muscles, number three and four lumbricals (the lumbricals nearest the hypothenar eminence) and *all the interossei.* Weakness of the lumbricals in median and ulnar nerve lesions leads to hyperextension at the metacarpo-phalangeal (MP) joints and begins the clawing (main en griffe) posture which is completed by flexion at inter-phalangeal (IP) joints, due to contracture of the flexors. The MEDIAN nerve enters the hand, passing under the flexor retinaculum and supplies the THENAR eminence and the two adjacent lumbricals.

Wasting of the small muscles of the hand

Observation *alone* before any more examination can localise the site of the lesion.

Look at the dorsum of the hand.
(1) Is there a LOCAL CAUSE? – The deformities of rheumatoid arthritis or terminal inter-phalangeal joint arthropathy (psoriasis).
(2) Is there a LOCAL CLUE? – Burns (syringomyelia), fasciculation (motor neurone disease).

Turn the hand over.
(1) Is the wasting UNILATERAL? – Suggesting a lesion below the neck and into the arm.
(2) Is the wasting BILATERAL? – Suggesting a lesion in the neck – *or* a peripheral neuropathy.
(3) Is it SYMMETRICAL affecting thenar and hypothenar eminences or is it ASYMMETRICAL affecting one or other, that is, is it of median or ulnar in distribution?

Look at the eyes.
Is there a Horner's syndrome present? That places the lesion in the lower chord of the brachial plexus (C8–T1).

Look at the face.
(1) If the wasting is thenar is there acromegaly or myxoedema?
(2) Is there frontal balding, cataract and sterno-mastoid wasting? – dystrophia myotonica.

Look at the feet.
Have they pes cavus? That would suggest peroneal muscular atrophy (the hands are involved late). Is there unilateral or bilateral foot drop? Then motor neurone disease or polyneuritis is the diagnosis.
In a matter of seconds important clues have been detected.
The shape of the hand depends:
(1) On wasting, soft tissue overgrowth or bony deformity.
(2) On posture due to muscle imbalances which may be fixed or tetanic.

411

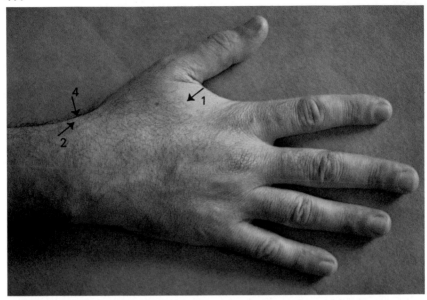

412

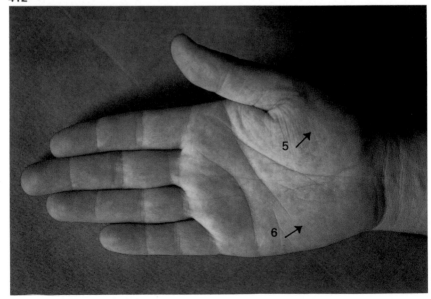

411 & 412 *The normal hand* Change due to habits (smoking, nail biting) and occupations may be seen. It has no soft tissue swelling, normal nails, no thenar, hypothenar or inter metacarpal wasting, no trophic changes, pigmentations or abnormality of colour. Note the fullness produced by the first dorsal interosseus muscle between the thumb and index (1). It is supplied by the ulnar nerve from the palm. N.B. Do not describe muscle wasting at 2, the anatomical snuffbox – a depression bounded by two tendons. Extensor pollicis longus (3) and extensor pollicis brevis (4). The floor is formed by the scaphoid bone. The full muscle bulk of the thenar eminence mainly supplied by the median nerve. Abductor pollicis brevis (median nerve) (5) which is weak in carpal tunnel compression. The hypothenar muscles (6) – ulnar nerve. (See also **413**.)

413 *Wasting of the small muscles of the hand (diabetic neuropathy)* In the right hand the first dorsal interosseus is wasted (1) and there is hollowing between the metacarpals where the other interossei are wasted. Note minor Heberden's nodes of fingers which are incidental.

On the facts observed you have unilateral muscle wasting affecting the interossei supplied by T1 via the ulnar nerve. *(Sir William Heberden, 1710–1801, published 1802.)*

413

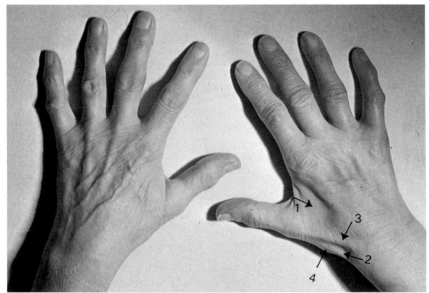

414 & 415 *Wasting abductor pollicis brevis (right)* Pain and paraesthesiae were relieved by carpal tunnel decompression. A cervical rib (*arrow*) was also present on the right side which could have accounted for her symptoms. There was no Raynaud's phenomenon and conduction studies demonstrated delay at the wrist.

WASTING OF THE HAND MUSCLES may be due to lesions at different levels. (1) *Anterior horn cells:* syringomyelia, polio, motor neurone disease. (2) *Anterior nerve root:* cervical spondylosis, cervical cord compression by tumour. (3) *Brachial plexus:* cervical ribs (**415**), injuries (**420**, **422**), bronchus (pancoast tumour, **438**). (4) *Trauma to peripheral nerve.*

414

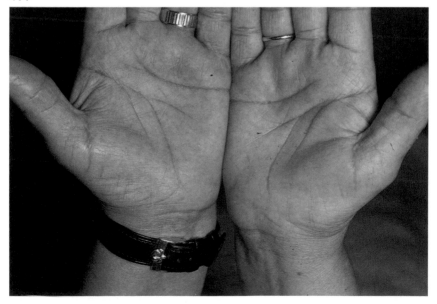

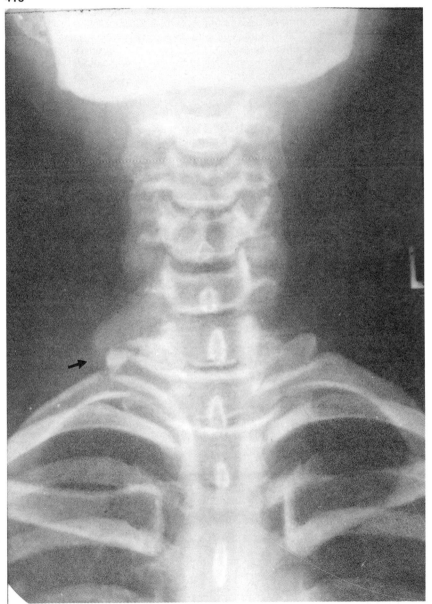

416 & 417 *Ulnar nerve palsy* The thumb, index and middle finger have normal posture (median normal). The ring and little finger are extended at the MP joint and flexed at the IP joint. The long extensors are acting without the stabilising effect of the ulnar lumbricals suggesting an ulnar nerve lesion. The first interosseus is wasted confirming that the ulnar nerve has been damaged (*arrow*). This is a partial main en griffe due to ulnar nerve palsy.

418 & 419 *The main en griffe (claw hand)* To produce the characteristic claw hand the small hand muscles must be paralysed either by a T1 lesion in the cord, which may be associated with a Horner's syndrome or by a median and ulnar nerve palsy in the hand. The lumbricals cannot act to oppose the actions of the long extensors of the fingers and hyperextension occurs at the MP joints and flexion at the IP joints due to the long flexors of the fingers. Note the hollowing in the metacarpal area of the dorsum of the hand and the flexion of the proximal IP joints with extension at the MP joint due to loss of lumbrical action, seen from the side (**418**), and wasting of all the interossei in figure **419**.

416

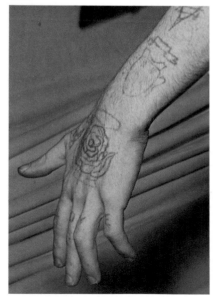

417

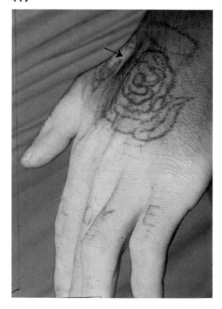

418

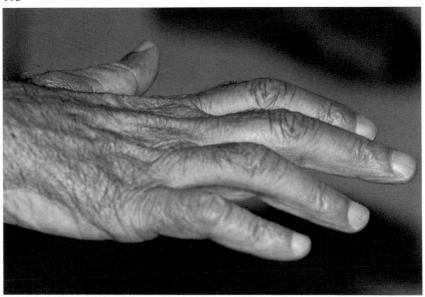

419

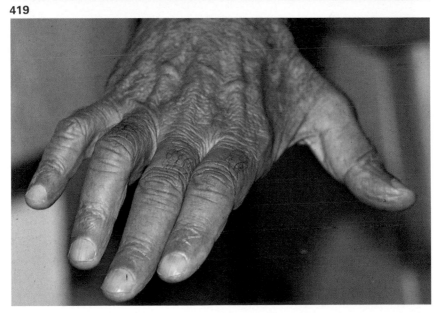

420 & 421 *Main en griffe* An extreme example of the effect of small muscle paralysis and contraction of paralysed long flexors of the fingers with unopposed action of the extensors without lumbrical balance. An ulnar and median nerve palsy due to a lesion of the lower chord of the brachial plexus due to a gunshot wound. The left palm shows loss of muscle bulk over the thenar and hypothenar eminence. There is extension at the metacarpal-phalangeal joints and flexion at the inter-phalangeal joints suggesting loss of action of the lumbricals. The long flexors of the fingers are contracted and the extensors of the fingers are extending the finger at the MP joint. (Note the atrophic change to the skin compared with the normal side.)

420

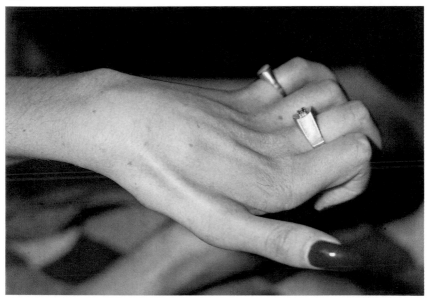

421

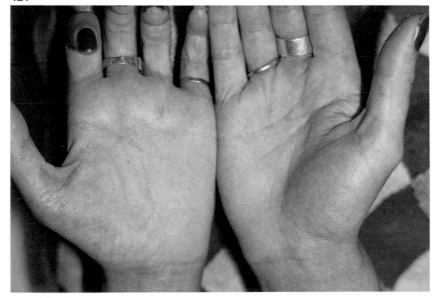

422

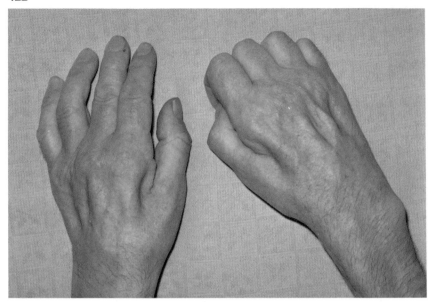

423

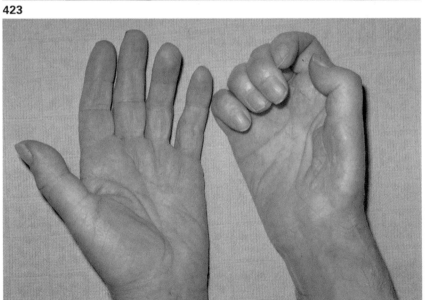

422–424 *Partial and complete wasting of the hand* A 50-year-old diabetic presents with wasting of the small hand muscles. Complicated anatomical deformity can be analysed if taken logically.

Dorsum of the hands (**422**). On the left: dorsal guttering = interosseous wasting = ulnar palsy. Extension/flexion/flex at MP/IP/IP joints of the ring and little fingers is the posture produced when the lumbricals are out of action. The 3rd and 4th lumbricals are supplied by the ulnar nerve. Thus: ulnar lesion – partial claw hand, but what is the level of the injury?

On the right: the guttering of interosseous wasting (ulnar lesion) plus flexed fingers suggest median and radial lesion (paralysis of forearm extensors) as well and put the level higher than the wrist.

Palm of the hands (**423**). On the left: confirms hypothenar wasting (ulnar palsy). In a diabetic it could therefore be a mononeuritis.

On the right: thenar and hypothenar wasting (therefore ulnar, radial, AND median nerve palsy). The final contracted hand.

Elbow (**424**). Confirms extensive wasting of the right forearm (ulnar, median and radial nerves affected), due to a branchial plexus injury. BUT: diabetic neuropathy must be questioned in view of the scar at the left elbow (*arrow*) of an ulnar nerve transposition.

424

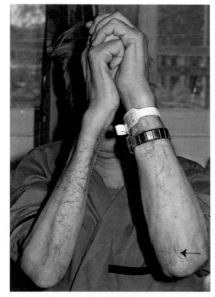

425 & 426 *Radial nerve palsy, wrist drop* The cardinal feature of a radial nerve palsy is wrist drop due to paralysis of the extensors of the wrist and fingers. The area of sensory loss covers the anatomical snuffbox.

425

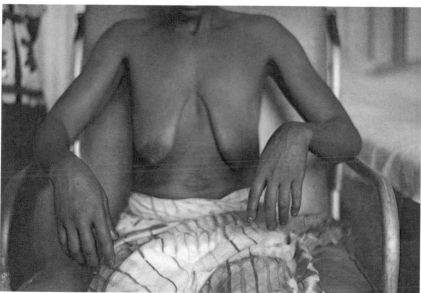

426

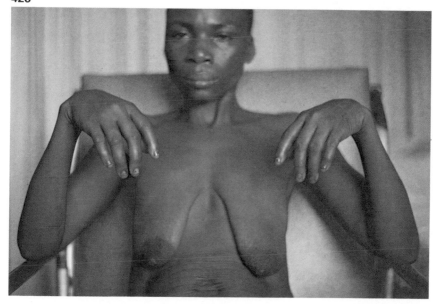

427 *Erb's paralysis C56* The arm hangs by the side of the forearm pronated and the fingers flexed into the 'waiter's tip' position. There is no voluntary movement of the arm: the fingers are spared. It is due to excess neck stretching at birth, usually in breech presentation, affecting the C56 roots. *(Wilhelm Heinrich Erb, 1840–1921, described 1874.)*

428 *Congenital contracture of the fingers* It is a common deformity apparent from birth, unrelated to nerve palsy, sometimes associated with congenital nystagmus. It has no neurological significance.

429 *Tetany, the main d'accoucheur* So-called 'obstetrician's hand', the posture is due to tetany of the muscles. It is seen in situations with a low ionized calcium – overbreathing, hypocalcaemia – it is brought out by applying a tourniquet in the form of a sphygmomanometer to the arm. It was first noted by Trousseau when a patient being bled for a rheumatic condition developed tetany when the arm bandage was applied to the arm. Here the patient has hypoparathyroidism and tetany was brought out by performing Trousseau's test. The colour change in the palm is due to the application of henna. *(Armand Trousseau, 1801–1867.)*

427

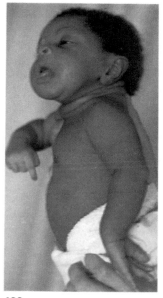

428

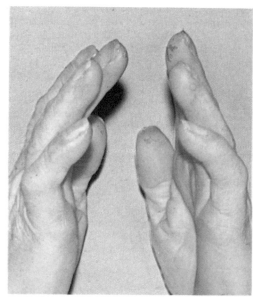

429

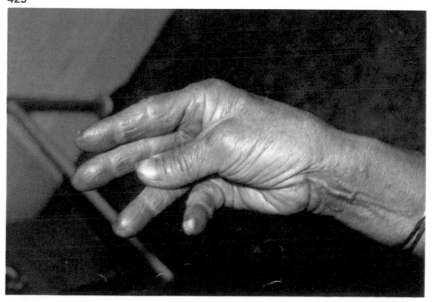

430–433 *Rheumatic chorea affecting the left side (5-second intervals)*
Involuntary varying movements when asked to hold the arm still and
outstretched. Purposeless co-ordinated writhings with twitches and grimaces.
Note the flexion of the finger, deviation of the head and pronation of the
hand.

Abnormal postures may be static (preceding plates) or acute and con-
stantly changing (**430**).

Tremors, both fine and coarse, do not lend themselves to still photography.
These involuntary, repetitive, rhythmic movements may be fine (felt more
easily than seen) or coarse and obvious. (1) Benign familial tremor – marked
when the hands are outstretched and often disappears at the essential part of
the movement; (2) Senile tremor; (3) Cerebellar intention tremor – brought
out by movement and increasing terminally – similar tremor occurs in toxicity
due to heavy metals, alcohol and drugs; (4) Extrapyramidal tremor
(Parkinson's disease) – increased by stress, emotion and movement; (5)
Anxiety – fine or coarse, present at rest, increased by movement, often
associated with tachycardia and clammy skin; (6) Thyrotoxicosis – fine,
constant; (7) Liver disease – the liver flap – wing flapping movement.

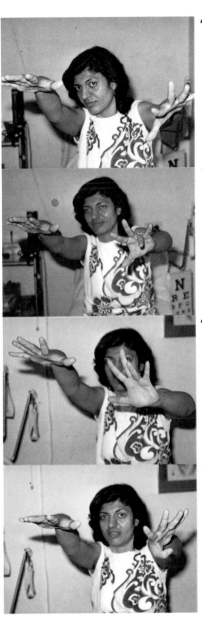

430   0 seconds

431   5 seconds

432   10 seconds

433   15 seconds

434 & 435 *Oedema of the hand (hemiplegia)* The right hand is swollen due to disuse oedema (**434**). X-ray of such an arm after a long period of time will show the appearance of disuse osteoporosis (**436**). Compare this hand with the fat meaty hand of the female acromegalic who has spatulate fingers and an excess of soft tissue (**435**).

434

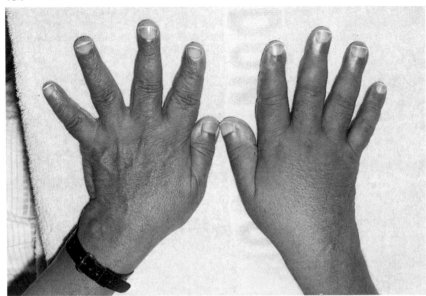

435

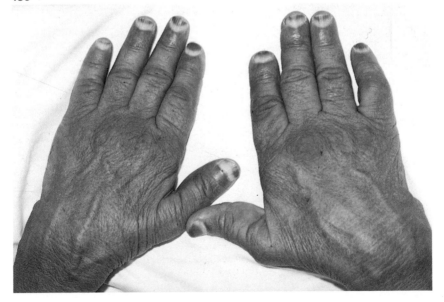

436 & 437 *Hemiplegia – osteoporosis* This is the picture of a right hemiplegia. This x-ray shows cystic areas affecting the humerus – the appearance of disease osteoporosis; the important points being the sclerotic margins to the cysts and the fact that the ribs are not affected. Similar changes affect the leg. The area in the square is enlarged below.

Figure **436** is very common and it may be mistaken, at first sight, for multiple myelomatosis and particularly if you are told the patient was old, febrile, with a raised sedimentation rate and pneumonia. The first diagnosis then offered is invariably multiple myelomatosis which is one thing it does not look like, an example of association of ideas (high ESR and bone lesions) and non critical observation. (In myeloma the bone lesions are clear cut without any sclerosis at the edges, so called 'punched out' lesions, **437**.)

438 *The simian hand (1st thoracic root invaded by carcinoma)* Wasting of the thenar and hypothenar eminence produces a flat palm with loss of opposition. The simian hand can be due to bilateral ulnar and median nerve lesions in a peripheral neuropathy, to dystrophia myotonica or to a central T1 root or chord lesion.

436 A

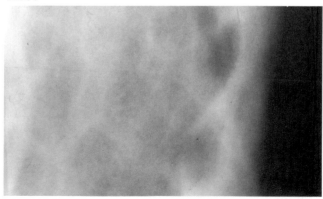

436 B

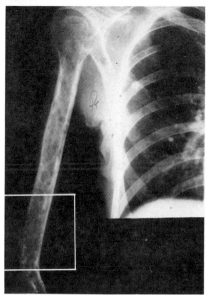

437

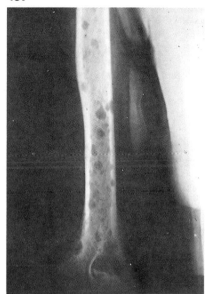

438

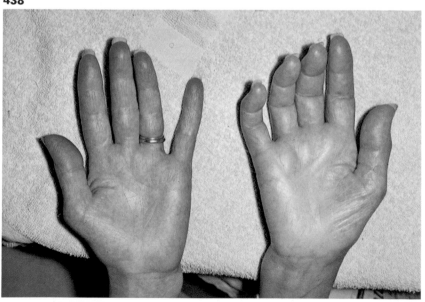

439–444 *Dupuytren's contracture of the palm* The series of six plates shows the development of the contracture from its earliest puckering of the skin through to complete tethering of the finger into the palm. The male preponderance is lost after the age of 60 years when the frequency is 20% of the population with an increased incidence in alcoholics, cirrhotics and epileptics. There may be a relationship with chronic trauma. Alcohol and barbiturates (epileptics) are both enzyme inducers and the effect on the liver and its reaction may be the common factor in the aetiology.

439, palmar erythema (liver palms), very early Dupuytren's contracture in a male alcoholic with cirrhosis. The moist palm reflects anxiety at imminent liver biopsy.

440, as the fascia contracts the palm skin puckers.

441, gradually the fingers flex at the metacarpo-phalangeal joint of the 4th ring and little fingers. Note the nicotine staining and the amputation: though irrelevant here, always note the additional signs for they may have a bearing on the analysis of a short case.

442–444, these three plates show the puckering produced in the skin (*arrow*) by the taut contracting fascia leading to eventual opposition between finger and palm. *(Guillaume Dupuytren, 1777–1835, described 1831.)*

439

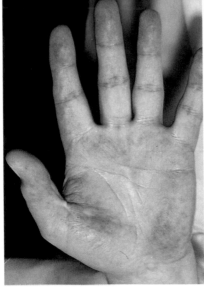

440

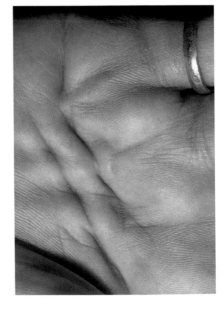

441

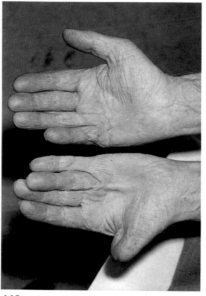

442

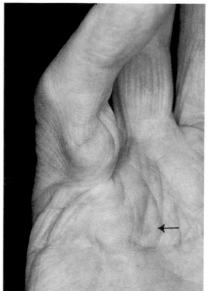

443

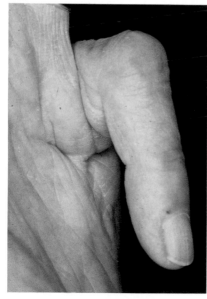

444

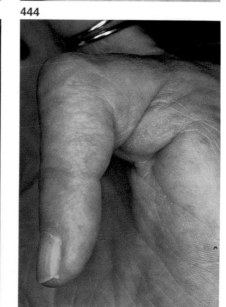

Raynaud's phenomenon

Characterised by episodic attacks of pallor followed by cyanosis and ending with vasodilation, sometimes accompanied by pain. It may be unilateral or bilateral and of all grades of severity.

Secondary Raynaud's may be due to disorders characterised by irritation of the sympathetic nerves, pathological alterations in small blood vessels or sludging and agglutination of red blood cells.

Causes

(1) Vascular – ergotism, emboli, arteriosclerosis.

(2) Neurogenic – cervical rib, costoclavicular compression, syringomyelia, polio.

(3) Collagen diseases – systemic lupus erythematosus, scleroderma, rheumatoid arthritis.

(4) Blood dyscrasias – cryoglobulinaemia, Hodgkin's disease.

(5) Trauma – *physical:* vibrations – pneumatic drillers; *thermal:* cold – fishmongers.

(6) Idiopathic – Raynaud's disease.

(7) Toxic – Vinyl chloride exposure.

445–447 *Raynaud's phenomenon* The initial pallor affecting one finger (**445**), changes over a few minutes to vasodilation (**446**). This is the earliest sign of Raynaud's phenomenon precipitated by cold. *(A G Maurice Raynaud, 1834–1881, described 1862.)*

445

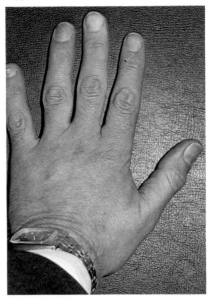

446

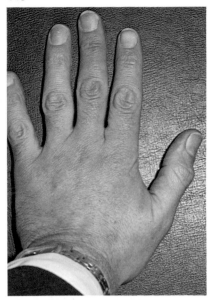

447

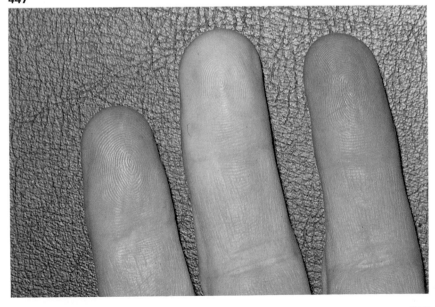

448 *Raynaud's disease* Idiopathic Raynaud's phenomenon (termed Raynaud's disease) in a young female. Severe vasoconstriction leading to gangrene of the right index and left middle finger with trophic changes affecting other fingers is rare. A cervical rib may produce a picture like this but bilateral gangrene is more often seen in emboli, ergotism or collagenosis. Burns in syringomyelia usually affect the lateral fingers.

449 *Raynaud's phenomenon* Affecting the right, middle and index fingers, which are paler than the other fingers. Note the wasting of the first dorsal interosseus (ulnar nerve) which suggests a T1 lesion or a cervical rib as a cause for the phenomenon.

450 *Raynaud's phenomenon (idiopathic)* The palmar surface of the same hands at a slightly later stage in the evolution of colour change, the index and middle fingers of the right hand have now taken on a blue tinge before finally reverting to normal. Note very slight wasting over abductor pollicis brevis in the right hand (*arrow*). Apart from that there are no abnormal physical signs.

451 *Raynaud's disease* Late result of Raynaud's disease progressing to gangrene in lupus erythematosus.

452 *Cervical rib* A rudimentary cervical rib may be seen as a pointed addition to the transverse process and suggests the presence of a fibrous band completing the rudimentary rib. This fibrous band may give rise to compression symptoms, particularly if the brachial plexus is pre or post fixed.

448

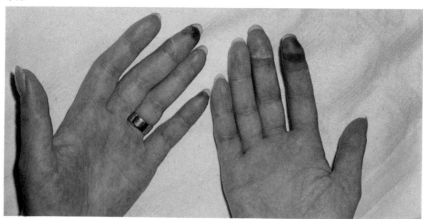

449

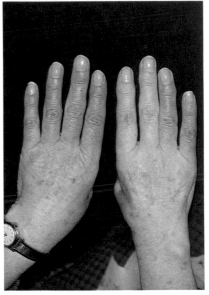

450

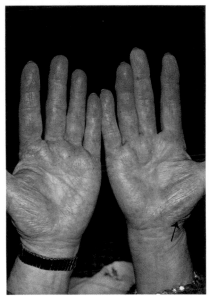

451

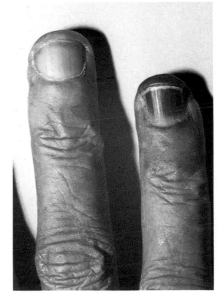

452

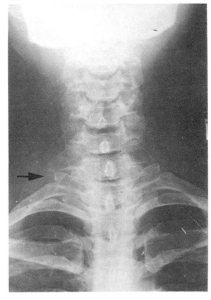

453 *Cervical rib* The classic cervical rib is obvious, provided one looks at the neck – it can often be felt as a bony resistance in the supraclavicular fossa.

454 *Raynaud's phenomenon secondary to scleroderma* The hand is shiny, the skin puffy and thickened. There are pale and red areas on the fingers. This woman had suffered from Raynaud's phenomenon for many years and had noted gradual stiffening and thickening of the skin of the fingers due to scleroderma.

455 & 456 *Scleroderma* This woman had Raynaud's phenomenon and then noted stiffness of the fingers and shininess of the skin – seen here by the high gloss on the skin in the sunlight.

453

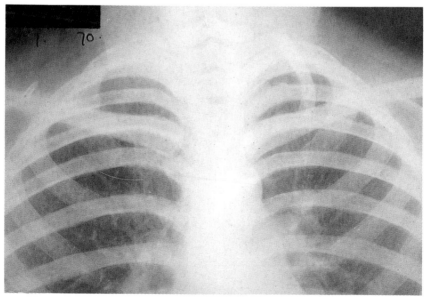

454

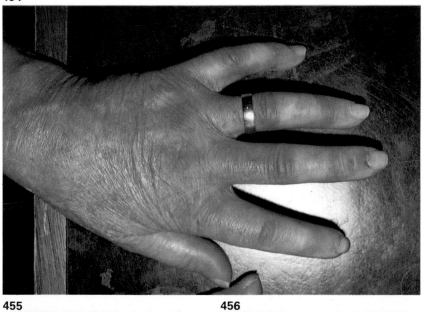

455

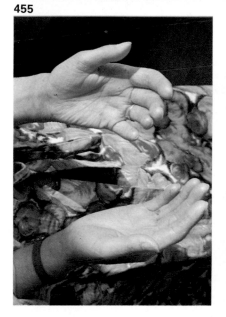

456

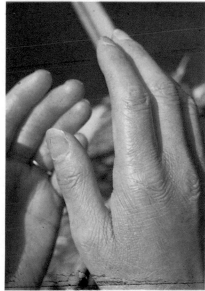

457 *Thromboangiitis obliterans (Buerger's disease)* A young male smoker with peripheral vascular disease affecting the feet *and* hands – terminal amputations have been performed for gangrene. This is an example of this disease which, in fact, may not be a distinct pathological entity but may purely be a rare manifestation of a common condition – arteriosclerosis. *(Leo Buerger, 1879–1943, described 1908.)*

458 *Venous obstruction in the hand* The left hand is red compared with the right and there is filling of the veins compared with the right hand (both held above the level of the heart). This woman had secondary deposits in the axilla from the carcinoma of the breast producing venous obstruction.

459 *Arterial obstruction (partial)* The hand is held above the level of the heart and the affected side blanches due to the arterial obstruction by emboli from a subclavian aneurysm.

457

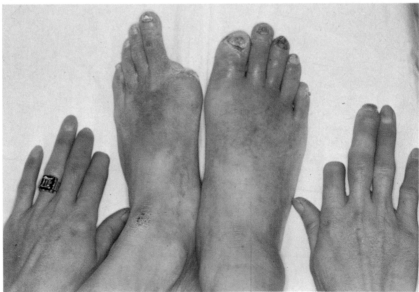

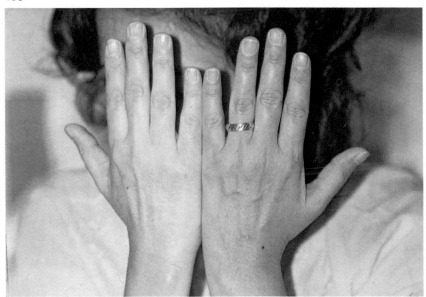

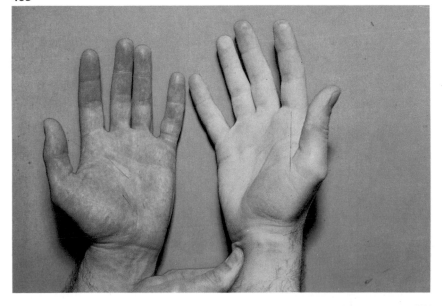

Swelling and deformity

460 *Rickets (dietary vitamin D deficiency)* There is bilateral swelling at the level of the lower radial epiphysis. A small umbilical hernia is present as well as swelling of the epiphysis at the lower end of the femora.

461 & 462 *Rickets* The clinically expanded epiphyseal junction is due to an increase in uncalcified osteoid at the widened and cupped epiphysis of the lower end of the radius. As it heals this x-ray reverts towards normal.

460

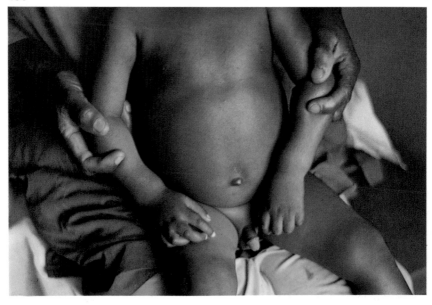

461

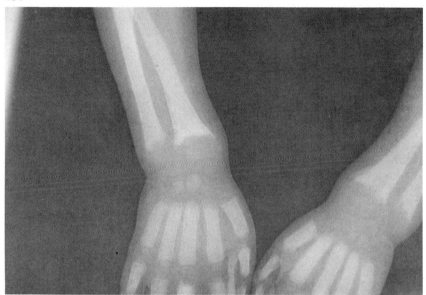

462

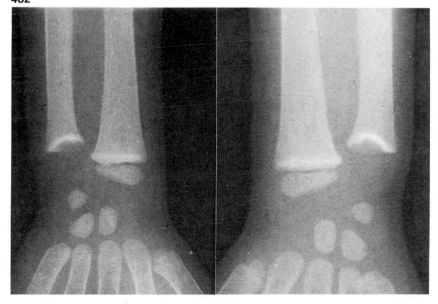

463–465 *Scurvy* Apart from the bleeding gums and the petechiae due to capillary fragility, vitamin C deficiency will produce defective calcification and sub-periosteal haematoma formation. This may be intensely painful – the patient, usually a small child, lies in a 'frog' position with the legs flexed and abducted at the hips. He may scream in anticipation of being moved. This x-ray of a Nigerian infant shows the flexed legs and the periosteal elevation due to the sub-periosteal haematoma.

The second and third x-ray shows the widening of the temporary calcification zone – 'the white line of scurvy' – and a translucent zone beneath the zone of temporary calcification. Note the defect in the spongiosa and cortex just below the epiphyseal plate (1) – the 'corner' sign of scurvy. Later true spurs may form (2).

463

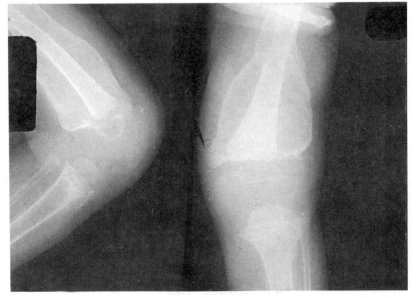

464

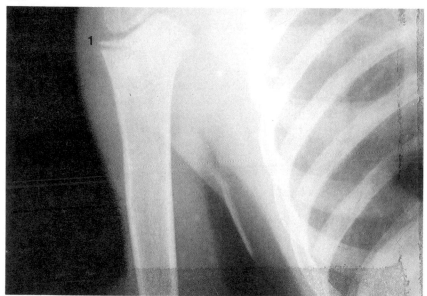

465

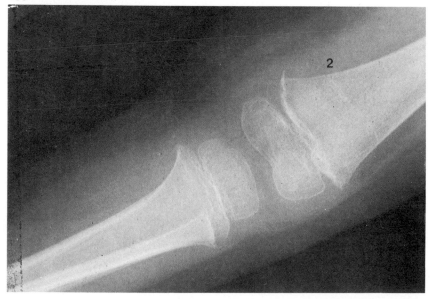

ARTHRITIS

When faced with the problem it is helpful to ask oneself: is it a mono or a poly arthritis? is it acute or chronic? which joints are affected, the small joints or the big joints? one large joint or one small joint? is it symmetrical or asymmetrical? is it migratory? does it leave a residual deformity and are there relapses and remissions? is the patient male or female? are there associated abnormalities in other systems?

With the answers to these questions a differential diagnosis can be formulated and it is then useful to have a pathological classification of possibilities on which to think *(Huskisson and Hart, 1975).*

Metabolic
gout
familial hypercholesterolaemia
ochronosis
Wilson's disease
pseudo gout

Mechanical and degenerative
osteoarthritis
traumatic arthropathies

The 'rheumatic diseases'
ankylosing spondylitis
palindromic rheumatism
polyarteritis nodosa
systemic lupus erythematosus
rheumatoid arthritis
polymyalgia rheumatica

Idiopathic
familial Mediterranean fever
sarcoidosis

Dietary
scurvy

Soft tissue syndromes – simulating arthritis
carpal tunnel compression
Dupuytren's contracture
tennis elbow

Infective
bacteria
viruses
parasites
fungi

Post infective
bacillary dysentery
Henoch-Schönlein purpura
rheumatic fever
Reiter's disease

Arthritis with disease of other major systems

Endocrinological
acromegaly
hyperparathyroidism
hypothyroidism
idiopathic hypoparathyroidism
thyroid acropathy

Haematological
haemophilia
leukaemia
sickle cell disease

Neurological
neuropathic

Gastroenterological
Crohn's disease
cirrhosis
Whipple's disease
ulcerative colitis

Dermatological
erythema multiforme
erythema nodosum
psoriasis

Neoplastic

Secondary bone disease
Paget's disease
rickets, etc

466 *Palindromic rheumatism (Gk running back, males = females)*
There is a swelling of the right wrist joint with filling out of the skin creases.
This 40-year-old man suffers from sudden, acute, recurrent attacks of pain
and swelling of one or both wrists and hands with a predilection for the
fingers, reverting entirely to normal after a few hours to two or three days.
This transitory inflammation was associated with little or no systemic reaction
or laboratory abnormality.
Differential diagnosis: (1) rheumatoid arthritis, (2) gout, (3) pseudo gout,
(4) systemic lupus erythematosus.
    He has not yet developed generalised arthropathy which may occur later in
palindromic rheumatism.

467 *Early acute rheumatoid arthritis* There is swelling of the proximal IP
joints particularly marked in the index, ring and middle fingers.

468 *Rheumatoid arthritis* Early but definite arthritis with swelling of the
proximal interphalangeal joint producing the characteristic spindle shape in
the index finger.

466

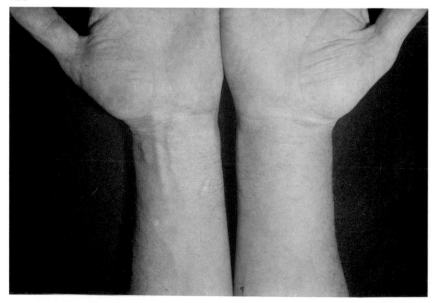

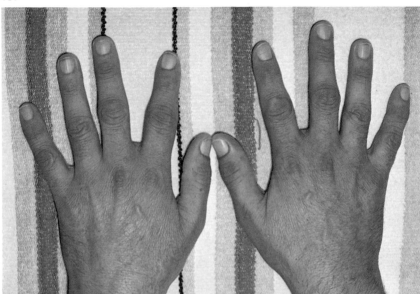

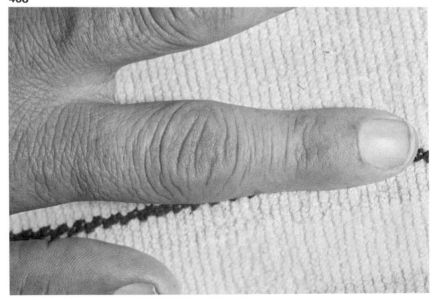

469 *Rheumatoid arthritis* X-ray of the preceding hand showing the earliest radiological changes of soft tissue swelling, corresponding to the clinical appearance, and peri articular osteoporosis.

470 *Polyarthritis, systemic lupus erythematosus* Swelling of all the IP joints of all the fingers with less obvious spindling compared with rheumatoid arthritis.

471 *Rheumatoid arthritis* A more advanced stage – less soft tissue swelling of the fingers and large rheumatoid nodules of the elbow. There is residual deformity with ulnar deviation of the fingers and incipient dislocation of the metacarpo phalangeal joint of the fifth finger.

Rheumatoid nodules may be seen on any bony prominence; the heel, elbows, occiput or in tendons.

469

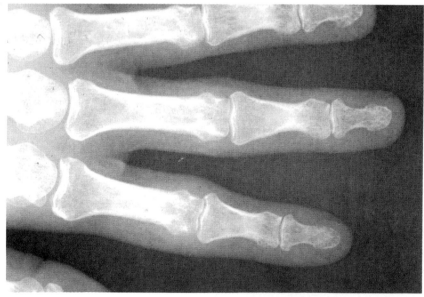

470

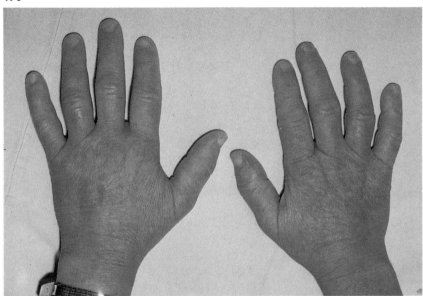

471

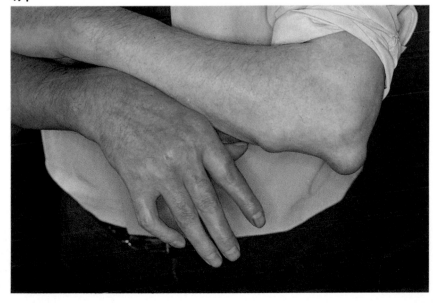

472 *Rheumatoid arthritis* A more advanced stage – joint swelling is less prominent and early small muscle wasting can be seen. Some flexion deformity has developed and there is subluxation, dislocation and consequent ulnar deviation of the fingers. Note: dislocation of the little finger at the MP joint secondary to joint damage.

473 *Rheumatoid nodule in the extensor tendon* When the nodule occurs at the junction with the tendons sheath 'triggering' may occur. These nodules may antedate the appearance of overt rheumatoid disease: they may be benign. They should not be confused with other lumps in the tendons.

474 & 475 *Benign nodule* The nodule is seen overlying the MP joint when the fingers are made into a fist and disappears on extension of the fingers.

472

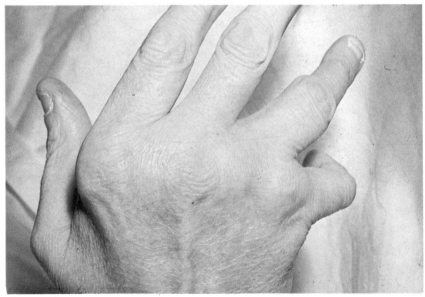

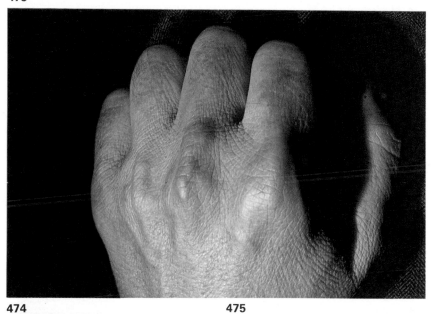

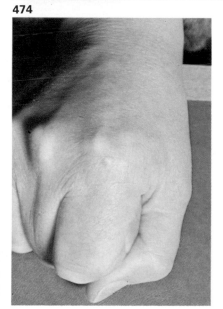

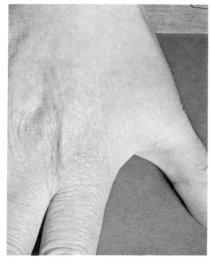

476 *Ganglion* A cystic degeneration of the joint capsule or tendon sheath, sometimes connecting with the joint, containing clear glairy fluid. The commonest site is the dorsum of the wrist. They can occasionally be 'emptied' into the joint, they transilluminate, are benign and frequently recur after excision.

477 & 478 *Ochronosis* The slate grey colour of the nodules in the extensor tendons shows through the skin. Compare these with the next plate where there is no such colour change (**479**). The pigment is derived from homogentisic acid (see **328**, the ear). Subsequent calcification in cartilage occurs producing this picture (**478**). It is associated with degenerative osteoarthritis.

479 *Tendon xanthomata* Lipid deposits in familial hypercholesterolaemia: other sites are the elbow, around the eyes and in the cornea. This man presented with angina; three other members of his family had xanthomata and hypercholesterolaemia.

480 *Down's syndrome, mongolism* The fingers are short, the hand spade-like and the little finger stubby. There may be some curvature of the little finger.

476

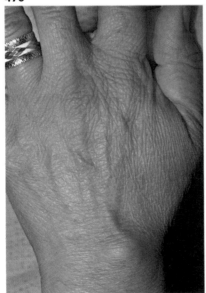

477

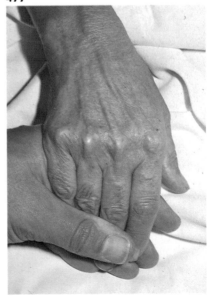

478

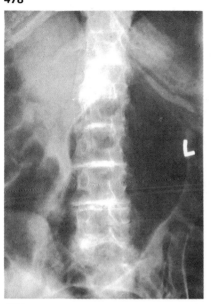

479

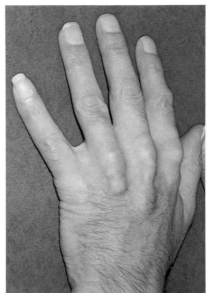

480

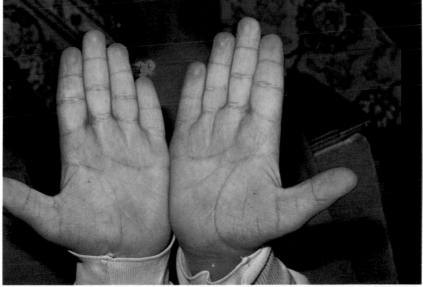

481 *Down's syndrome* The characteristic angle produced by the tri-radii (*arrows*) demonstrates the broadness and shortness of the palm. When the palm is short in the extreme a single transverse crease is present. *(John Langdon Haydon Down, London Hospital, 1828–1896, described 1866.)*

482 *Acromegaly* Female hand compared with a normal female of the same age. Note the broad spatulate fingers, the thickening and overgrowth of the soft tissues of the hand, particularly marked over the first dorsal interosseus.

483 & 484 *Acromegaly* The x-ray changes in the hand in acromegaly consist of (1) tufting, (2) an increase in joint space (cartilage) and (3) an increase in cortical bone thickness. Cortical bone thickness is well shown in these pictures. This produces loss of concavity in the shafts of the phalanges by virtue of bony ridges. Some lipping of the joint margins is present.

481

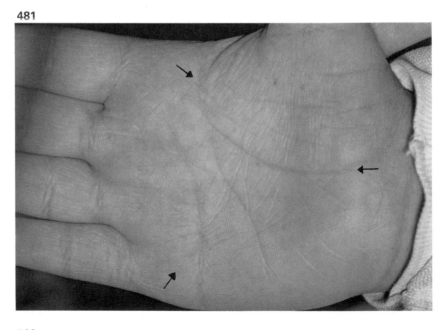

482

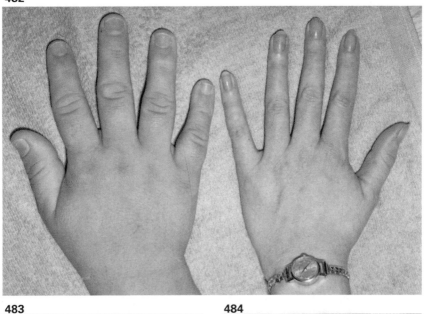

483

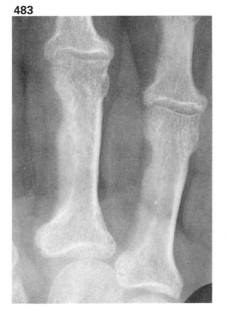

484

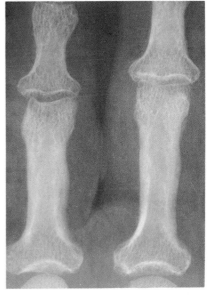

485 & 486 *Hyperparathyroidism* This woman complained of pains in the knees and was thought to have osteoarthritis. There was some osteoporosis and a little calcification in the cartilages (chondrocalcinosis). Ten weeks earlier she had caught her right hand in the car door and now noted a swelling which is easily seen. The x-ray demonstrates the underlying bone cyst and shows changes in the hands in hyperparathyroidism. (1) Osteoporosis, (2) bone cysts, (3) chondrocalcinosis, (4) sub-periosteal erosions and absorption of the tips of the terminal phalanges. The erosive changes are often seen in decreasing severity from index to little fingers and tend to be more marked on the radial side of each finger, possibly related to decreasing trauma on the fingers – index to little – in daily life.

487 *Haemochromatosis* The haemachromatotic arthropathy may affect the hand. Note the calcification in the cartilage at the MP joint of the fifth and ring fingers.

    The chondrocalcinosis would be typical of: (1) haemochromatosis; (2) pseudo-gout; (3) Wilson's disease; (4) hyperparathyroidism; (5) gout – rarely. These conditions should be excluded. It may also occur in ordinary degenerative joint disease.

488 *Dactylitis* The middle finger is swollen. There are no other abnormalities seen. Dactylitis may be acute or chronic, the acute variety may be related to trauma and inflammation, the chronic variety due to tuberculosis, syphilis and sarcoid. A relapsing variety of dactylitis is seen with recurrent bony infarcts in sickle cell disease. Swelling of the finger occurring in gout may be mistaken for dactylitis.

485

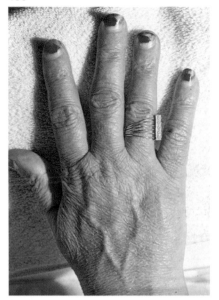

486

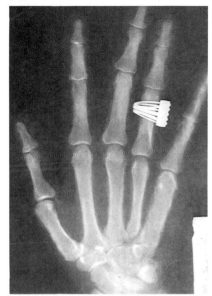

487

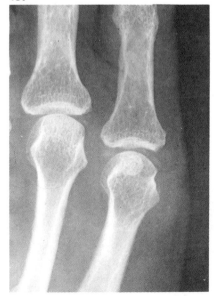

488

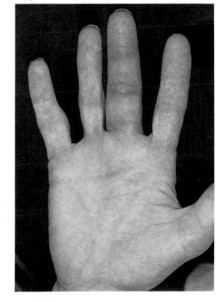

489 *Sickle cell dactylitis* Homozygous sickle cell disease often presents in small children with acutely swollen tender fingers due to a bone crisis in the phalanges. Subsequent infarction occurs.

490 *Sickle cell dactylitis* After the initial bone crisis infarction may occur, leading to shortening of the phalanx. This boy, age 16, had had recurrent bone crisis due to sickle cell disease, affecting the little finger at the age of four years.

491 *The hemiplegic hand (right hemiplegia)* Disuse of the hand will lead to dependant oedema of the fingers which give the superficial appearance of dactylitis. Compare it with the preceding and subsequent pictures.

492 *Sarcoidosis with bone cysts of the digits* The appearance of the digits is similar to a chronic dactylitis or oedema. The swelling is solid and the diagnosis may be confirmed clinically by looking for other signs – lupus pernio. The x-ray appearances are of bone cysts distending the cortex.

493 *Sarcoidosis (x-ray)* Bone cyst in the proximal phalanx of the foot distending the bone. Appearance may consist of: (1) circumscribed cysts; (2) soft tissue swelling; (3) calcification in soft tissues (hypercalcaemia).

489

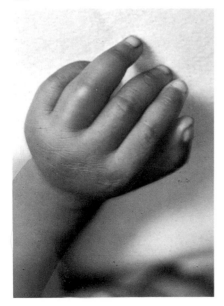

490

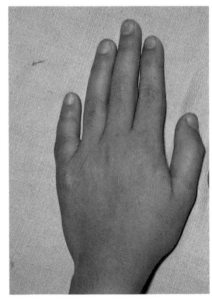

491

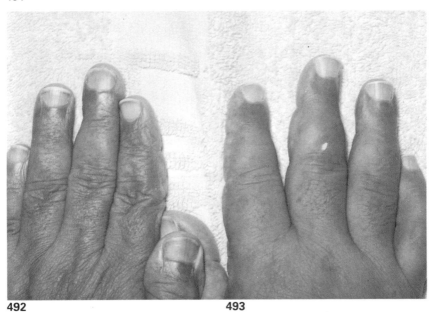

492

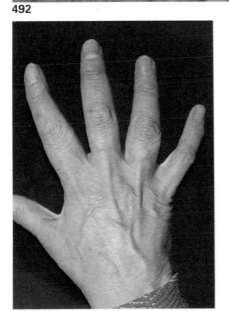

493

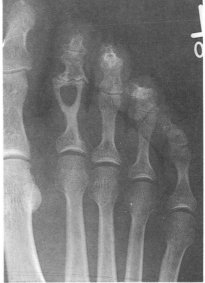

494 *Chronic gout* Tophi are present at the elbow, at the base of the thumb and in the fingers. Compare this with **471**, rheumatoid arthritis.

495 *Chronic tophaceous gout* Some of the tophi have ulcerated and discharged a creamy white substance which contains uric acid crystals.

496 *An ulcerated tophus*

497 *Gout* Tophi in chronic gout.

498 *Chronic tophaceous gout* The size of the tophii can be extreme and at first sight may mimic a rheumatic arthritic deformity.

494

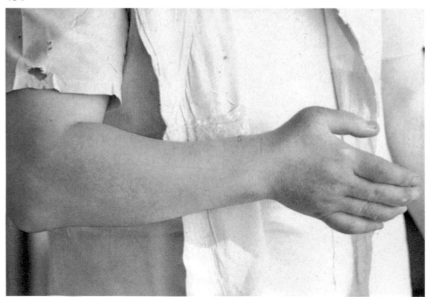

495

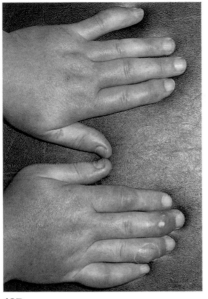

496

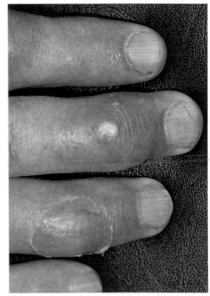

497

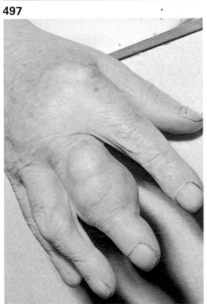

498

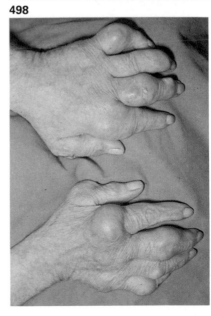

499 *Chronic tophaceous gout* Heberden's nodes are common and chronic tophaceous gout rare in the post menopausal female. This woman has gout and the uric acid material can be seen shining through the reddened skin.

The differential diagnosis of all finger tip swellings is from Heberden's nodes which are *commonplace* manifestations of osteoarthritis.

500 *Heberden's nodes* Bony protuberance affecting the base of the terminal phalanx, usually painless, occasionally aching. It occurs more commonly in women than in men. In the male it is often associated with a more generalised form of osteoarthrosis. The differential diagnosis from other swellings of the terminal phalanx is covered in the following plates which are compared alongside pictures of Heberden's nodes. *(William Heberden, 1710–1801, Physician to Dr Samuel Johnson, described posthumously 1802.)*

501 *Heberden's nodes (male)* Note the characteristic double bump on the dorsal aspect of the joint. There is no deformity.

502 *Osteoarthritis, hands* This woman has extensive Heberden's nodes coupled with later osteoarthritic changes in the fingers with some deformity, particularly of the right index and middle finger, typical of advanced osteoarthritis of the hands.

499

500

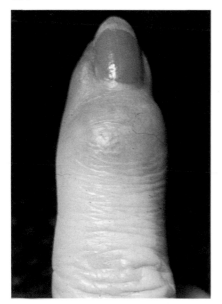
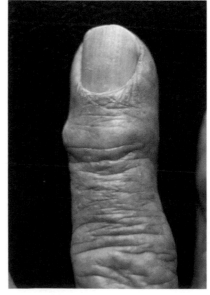

501

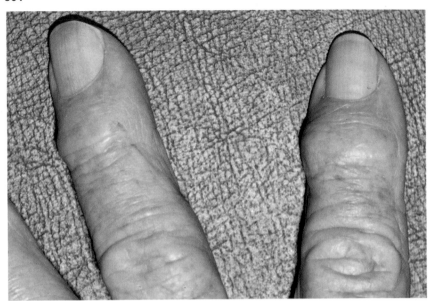

502

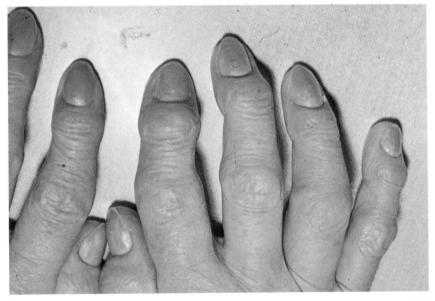

503 *Psoriasis of the nail* The earliest sign, of pitting, and one easily overlooked, may precede or coexist with the psoriatic arthropathy.

504 *Psoriatic arthritis* Swelling at the terminal interphalangeal joint is present; compare with the double bump of Heberden's nodule (**505**). There is some ridging of the nail and characteristic pitting. This is a typical picture of psoriatic arthropathy.

505 *Swelling of the terminal IP joint, Heberden's node* Some nail beading, which is an ageing phenomenon, is seen. There is deviation of the terminal phalanx of the right side of the finger, but there are no changes suggestive of psoriasis and the characteristic double bump of Heberden's node is visible.

503

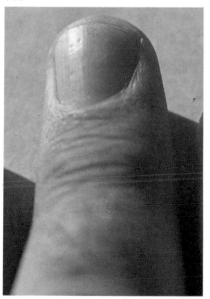

504

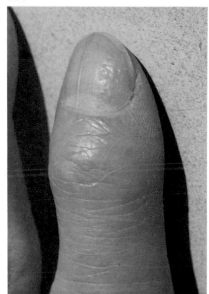

505

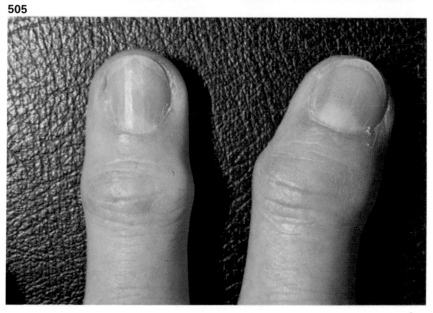

506 & 507 *Hypertrophic pulmonary osteoarthropathy* Swelling of the terminal phalanx of the fingers is present but there is marked curvature of the nail with loss of the normal obtuse angle at the nail fold. This is gross clubbing. The patient complained of pain in the joints of the extremities. On the x-ray periosteal bone reaction can be seen on the metacarpal of the thumb (*arrow*). Periosteal reaction is much more common on the bones of the forearms and legs. This patient had bronchiectasis but by far the commonest cause is a carcinoma of the bronchus.

508 & 509 *Psoriatic arthropathy* The full blown picture. The terminal IP joint swelling can be seen in the little and ring fingers. There is nail ridging, the pitting is visible in the close up and the plaque of psoriasis is seen in the bottom right hand corner on the wrist.

506

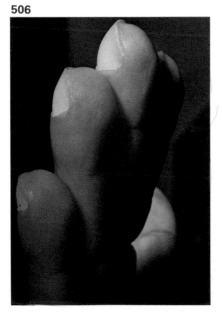

507

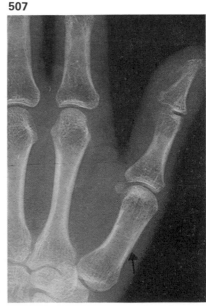

508

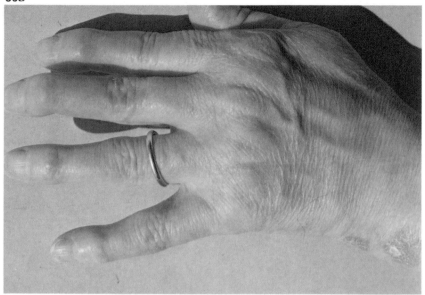

509

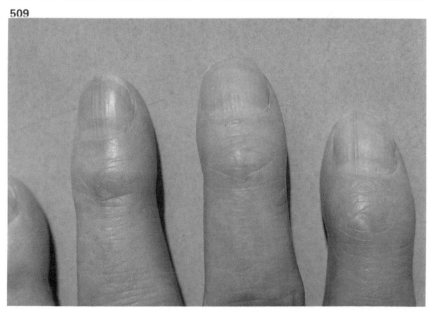

THE NAILS

510 & 511 *Normal nails* Anterior view and lateral view. Note the smooth surface of the nail with occasional white flecks. The angle the nail makes with the axis of the finger is less than 180°. Compare this with the clubbed finger (**512**) where the nail angle with the axis of the finger is now greater than or equal to 180°.

512 *Clubbing of the fingernails (minimal)* On the right the abnormal, and on the left the normal nail. The earliest sign of clubbing is a loss of the obtuse angle between the nail and the dorsum of the finger which goes past 180°. The nail bed is spongy and there is marked lateral curvature of the nail.

513 *Clubbing of the fingernail (minimal)* This is associated with cardio-respiratory disorders, alimentary tract disorders and rarely thyroid disease.
   Cardio-respiratory disorders: (1) lung disease – chronic inflammation, bronchiectasis; pulmonary fibrosis; carcinoma bronchus; pulmonary hypertension. (2) cyanotic heart disease.
   Alimentary tract disorders: (1) hepatic cirrhosis – clubbing proportioned to finger blood flow except in primary biliary cirrhosis. (2) malabsorption states – Crohn's disease, chronic diarrhoea, purgative addicts.

510

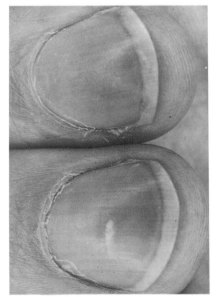

511

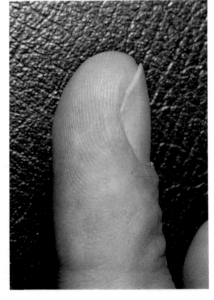

512

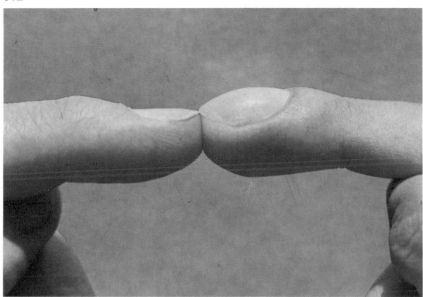

513

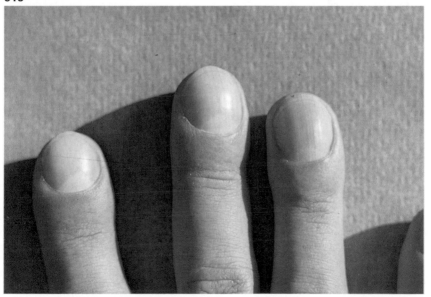

514 & 515 *Clubbing of the fingers (gross)* A patient with cirrhosis of the liver. Not only are the fingernails clubbed but the end of the fingers have a drum stick appearance, this may be extreme (**515**).

516 *Heberden's nodes for comparison*

517 *Clubbing of the fingernails (gross)* Bacterial endocarditis. A bulbous finger tip with beaking of the fingernail.

514

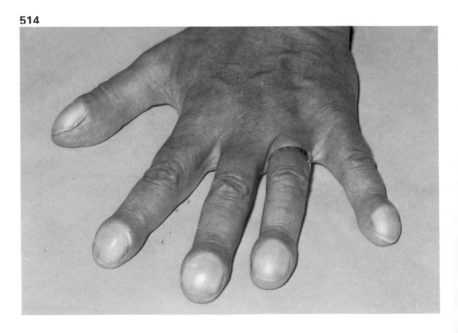

515

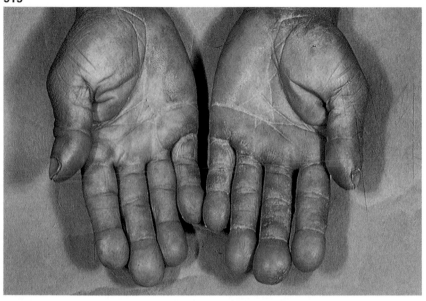

516

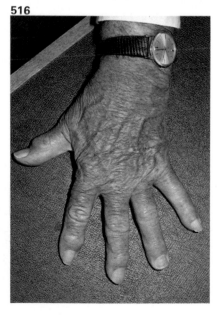

517

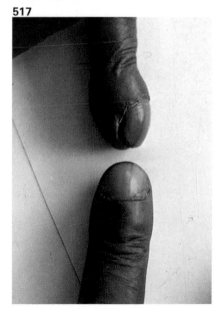

518 & 519 *Koilonychia* A flattened 'spoon-shaped' nail. The causes are (1) iron deficiency (Paterson-Brown Kelly/Plummer-Vinson syndrome: dysphagia – post cricoid web; anaemia – iron deficient; koilonychia), (2) development anomaly, (3) in infancy, (4) liver disease. *(Donald Rose Paterson, 1863–1939, described 1919; Adam Brown Kelly, 1865–1941, described 1919; Henry Stanley Plummer, 1874–1937, described 1912; Porter Paislery Vinson, born 1890, described 1919.)*

520 *Early koilonychia* When it is not so pronounced it presents as brittle flat nails.

521 *Pallor of the nailbed* The nails are a good site for comparing normal and abnormal and judging the degree of anaemia present. The lower set of nails is normal. Small white flecks in the nail may be related to trauma to the nailbed when the nail was growing. The nail is translucent and shows the pinkness of the capillary bed beneath. The upper nails are also translucent but demonstrate pallor of the nailbed. The haemoglobin of the patient was 6g%.

522 *The nails in chronic renal failure* The brown half moon of chronic renal failure, (the half and half or in this case the quarter and three-quarter nail). This is compared with the normal nail on the right. A white nail may be seen in chronic hypoalbuminaemia.

518

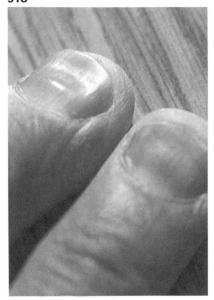

519

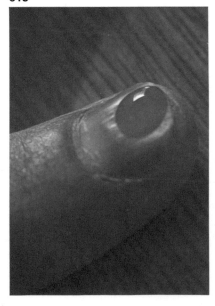

520

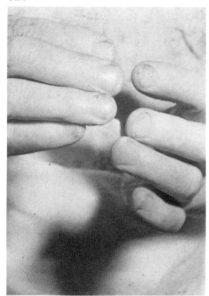

521

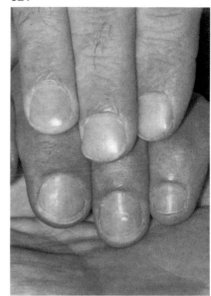

522

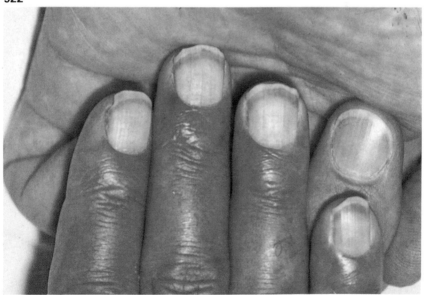

523 *Splinter haemorrhage* These changes have by tradition been associated with subacute bacterial endocarditis, but the commonest cause is trauma. They do however occur in many medical conditions ranging from severe rheumatoid arthritis and malignant neoplasia to psoriasis, dermatitis and fungus infections. They are therefore rather a non-specific sign and are of little value in diagnosis.

524 *Onycholysis* Separations of the nail from the nailbed. This occurs in many conditions and is one of the features of psoriasis, fungus infections, drug eruptions, poor circulation, Raynaud's phenomenon and trauma.

525 & 526 *Psoriasis* The earliest sign is pitting on the nail surface. The change may occur before the psoriasis is apparent elsewhere. Occasionally the pits are regular and form lines across the nails. Pitting may also be seen in dermatitis and chronic paronychia and it may also occur with other diseases such as alopecia areata. The pits are due to retention of nuclei in parts of the nail keratin which are then weaker than the surrounding normal keratin and are shed leaving pits on the surface. Onycholysis or separation of the bed also occurs as often as pitting. It is usually partial. There is usually a yellow margin visible between the pink and normal nail and a wide separated part. Gross abnormalities of the nail plate also occur and the nail grows deformed. The thickening and yellow colour change in onycholysis is well seen in **524**.

523

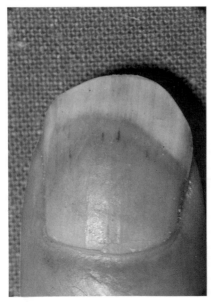

524

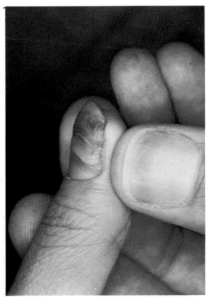

525

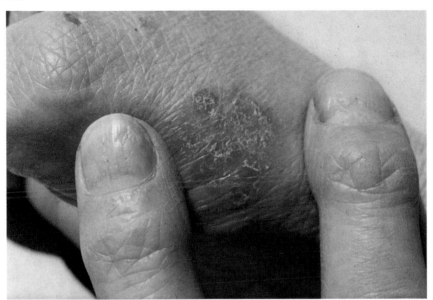

526

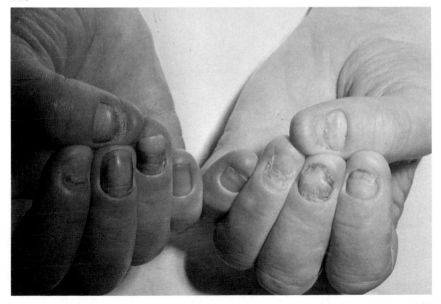

527 & 528 *Ridging/beading of the nail* In **527** a normal nail, and in **528** a nail showing ridging and beading. This is said to occur more often in rheumatoid arthritis than in normal people and it is more common in old age than in youth.

529 *White marks on the nails* May occur in: (1) minor trauma; (2) chronic arsenic poisoning; (3) chronic liver disease; (4) hypoalbuminaemia; (5) chronic renal disease; (6) Hodgkin's disease.

530 *Beau's lines* Transverse ridges in the nail occur with the slowing of nail growth during a debilitating illness, infectious fever or other serious upset. Growth picks up again after the illness. Local interference with blood supply can produce a similar effect.
   This patient had smallpox two months before this photograph was taken.
(Honoré Simon Beau, 1806–1865, described 1846.)

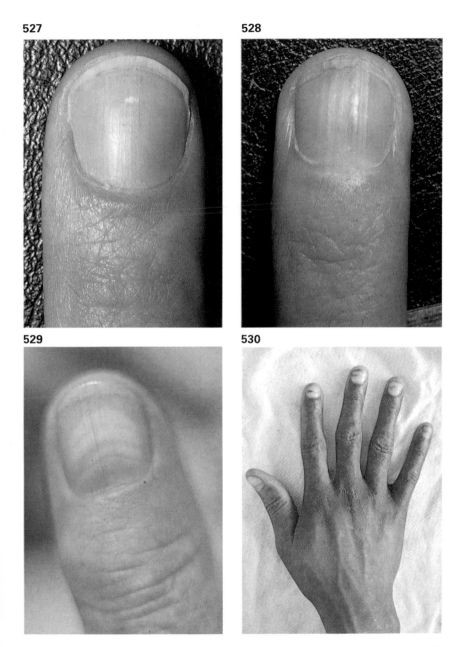

531 *Beau's lines* Observations: (1) Beau's lines are unilateral; (2) the upset occurred 5mm of growth ago (nail grows about 0.1–0.2mm a day); (3) the patient stopped putting henna on both feet at that time – she did not have any interest in her appearance; (4) the hair grows sparsely on the foot with Beau's lines.

Deductions: the patient had an episode of acute arterial insufficiency which has left the *left* leg (Beau's lines) ischaemic (hair growth depressed) about six weeks ago (5mm growth). She herself was also ill (cosmetically uninterested).

532 *Hyperkeratosis of the palms* The commonest cause is manual labour. This may be a congenital genetically determined disorder of hyperkeratosis of the hand and feet associated in some instances with an increased instance of oesophageal carcinoma. It can also occur with an ectodermal defect and premature shedding of the teeth in youth – the Papillon Lefeuvre syndrome (**360**). It also occurs in arsenic poisoning, in psoriasis, secondary to physical labour and friction, and as a toxic effect of certain drugs. Secondary hyperkeratosis of the hands and feet may be seen in syphilis and in Reiter's disease with keratodermia blennorrhagica. *(Hans Reiter, born 1881, described 1916.)*

531

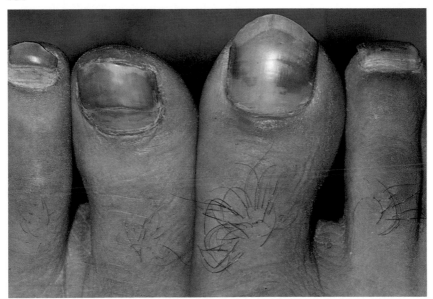

532

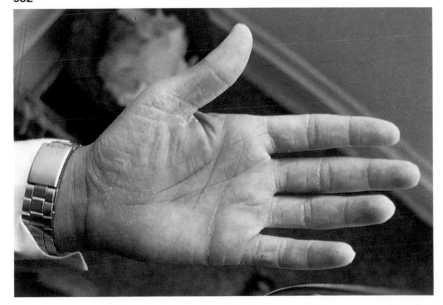

The Neck

533 *Torticollis* Congenital torticollis secondary to contraction of the sterno-mastoid on the left side. There is facial asymmetry. A similar appearance may be due to ocular imbalance producing ocular torticollis.

534 *Short neck* This appearance should pose the questions (1) is it a Klippel-Feil syndrome? (2) is it really a webbed neck? – Turner's syndrome (XO chromosome) includes increased carrying angle at the elbow, amenorrhoea, and association with coarctation of the aorta. *(Henry Hubert Turner, born 1892, described 1938.)*

535 & 536 *Klippel-Feil syndrome* Congenital abnormality with fusion of some vertebrae of the cervical spine leading to an abnormally short neck. This may lead to pressure disturbances of the spinal cord or cervical nerve roots. *(Andre Feil, born 1884; Maurice Klippel, 1858–1942; described 1912.)*

533

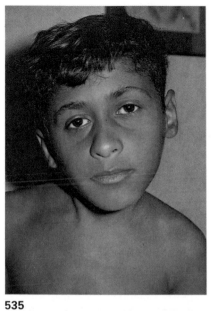

534

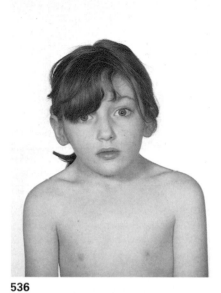

535

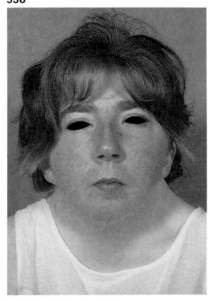

536

537 *Neck retraction* This may occur in inflammation of the meninges – meningitis, either acute or when long standing in tuberculous meningitis and in disorders of the basal ganglia. Spasmodic neck retraction occurs in tetanus. Neck retraction when associated with coma should always raise the possibility of undiagnosed tuberculous meningitis even when the diagnosis of a vascular accident seems obvious. In cases of severe raised intracranial pressure there may also be neck retraction.

538 *Neck retraction in tetanus*

539 *Lingual thyroid* The thyroid migrates from the branchial arch from which it is derived, along the thyroglossal track to take up its position in the neck. Failure of migration produces a lingual thyroid, failure of obliteration of the track may produce a thyroglossal cyst anywhere along the track or a sinus may persist at the skin.

540 *Ludwig's angina* Produces swelling of the neck, situated centrally. It is due to a spread from an infected tooth usually in the lower jaw. *(Wilhelm Friedrich von Ludwig, 1790–1865, described 1836.)*

541 *Cervical cellulitis* Another cause of swelling in the upper neck. It may be painful and tender and is usually related to a tooth infection.

537

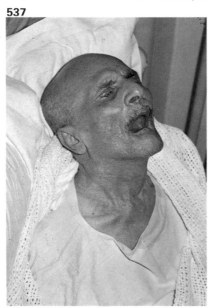

538

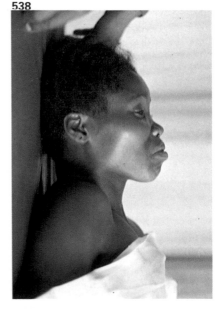

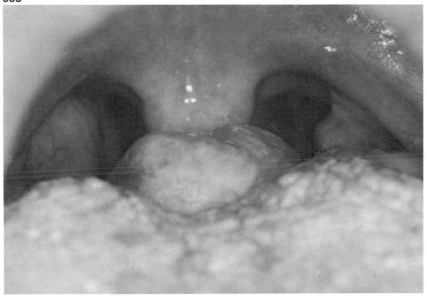

539

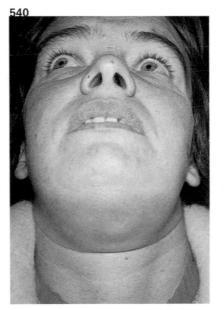

540

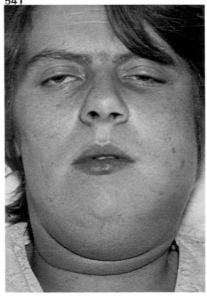

541

542 *Cat scratch disease* The essentials are: (1) lymphadenitis, one region; (2) sequel to an accidental skin injury, after a cat bite or scratch that could have been up to several weeks earlier; (3) granulomatous reaction in lymph node, secondary to presumed viral infection, which may suppurate.

543 *Lateral view enlarged sub-mental lymph node* It lies immediately anterior to the hyoid bone.

544 *Midline swellings* Enlarged sub-mental lymph node secondary to inflammation of the skin around the mouth. In this case the histology of the lymph node showed multiple granulomata without acid fast bacilli present. A sub-mental node lies in the midline and confusion may arise with aberrant thyroid tissue and a thyroglossal cyst.

545 & 546 *Thyroglossal cyst* This cyst is a remnant of the thyroglossal duct, the track along which the thyroid migrates. Failure of obliteration leads to cyst formation which may occur anywhere from the base of the tongue around the loop of the hyoid down to the base of the neck.

542

543

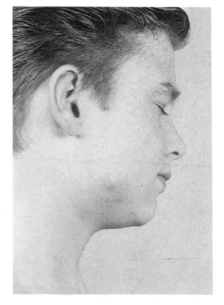
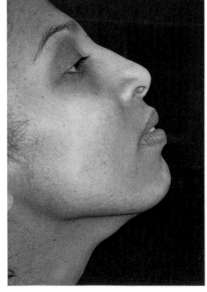

544

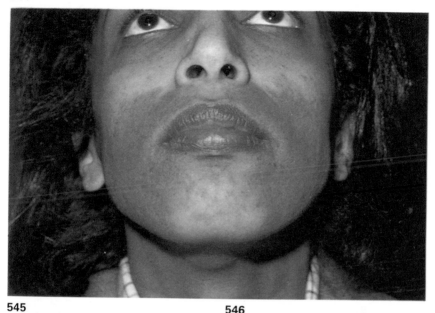

545

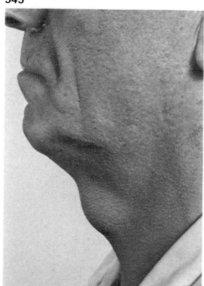

546

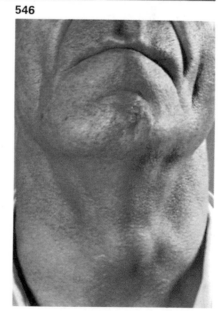

547 & 548 *Aberrant thyroid gland* The appearance of this central midline swelling is that of a thyroglossal cyst. However a scan of the neck showed that there was no other functioning thyroid tissue present. It is important before excising an apparent thyroglossal cyst to ensure that this is not the only thyroid tissue that the patient has.

549 *Sinus of thyroglossal duct* It can be seen that this is in the same position as the aberrant thyroid. Careful dissection up to the hyoid bone was necessary to remove it.

550 *Simple goitre* A fullness is seen in the anterior part of the neck.

551 & 552 *Goitre* On swallowing the goitre can be seen to move upwards. The lateral view shows the characteristic bi-lobed appearance of the enlarged thyroid gland.

547

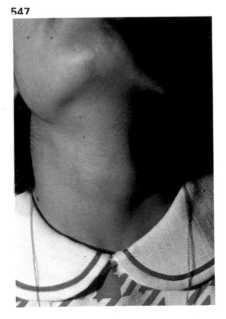

548

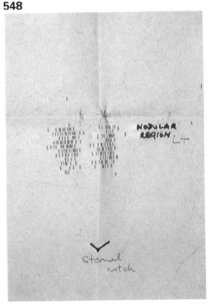

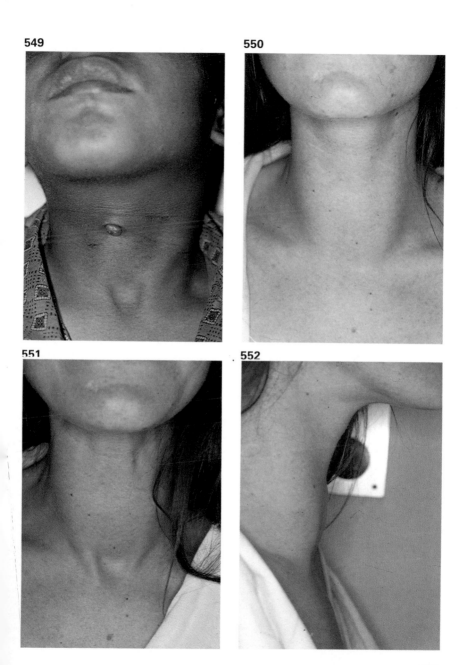

553 *Carcinoma thyroid* Greater enlargement of the gland is shown in this case of carcinoma of the thyroid, the goitre having been present for many years. The anatomy is still preserved.

554 *Lateral view of enlarged thyroid* Enlarged thyroid due to carcinoma of the thyroid. A characteristic of swellings in the thyroid is movement on swallowing.

555 & 556 *Thyroid nodule* Medial or lateral nodules can be shown to be part of the gland as they move with it on swallowing.
   In these pictures a central nodule moves up on swallowing (**556**).

553

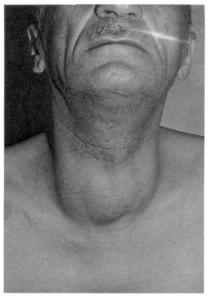

554

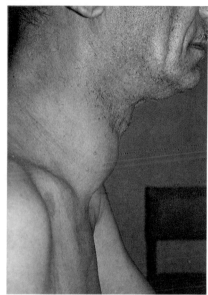

555

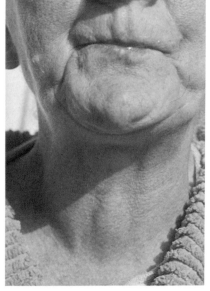

556

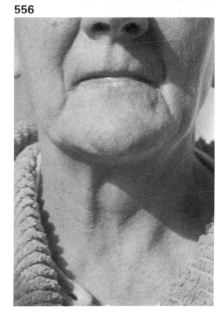

Mediastinal obstruction

This syndrome is due to obstruction to venous flow in the superior mediastinum. This may be caused by a tumour, usually bronchogenic carcinoma or enlarged glands in a lymphoma, pressing on the great veins and it is this pressure that produces the physical signs in the distribution of the superior vena cava. When the trachea is pressed upon, difficulty in breathing arises and pressure on the lymphatics produces further oedema.

The physical signs therefore are: (1) plethora; (2) injection of the eyes; (3) cyanosis; (4) difficulty in breathing with stridor; (5) distended neck veins and distended veins under the tongue.

The spectrum of signs runs from the very earliest dilatation of the external jugular vein through to a blue, swollen face with extreme respiratory distress and is shown in **557–564**.

557 *Mediastinal obstruction* Malignant lymphoma with thyrotoxicosis. Early mediastinal obstruction is present. Notice the fullness of oedema over the anterior chest particularly over the sternum, and the dilated jugular vein in the right side of the neck. There is a fullness on the left side of the neck due to enlarged lymph glands, the eyes are shiny, there is slight lid retraction (compare with **558** after Carbimazole therapy).

558 *Mediastinal obstruction* After treatment with Carbimazole and radiotherapy for one week. The lid retraction is less marked. Venous obstruction is improving.

559 *Early mediastinal obstruction* This man had a bronchogenic carcinoma with pressure on the superior vena cava secondary to glandular enlargement. Note the scar in the sternal notch from mediastinoscopy and the early dilatation of the neck veins. A corneal arcus is present.

557

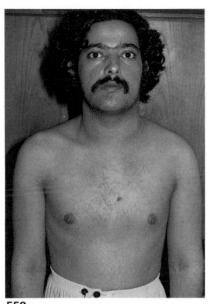

558

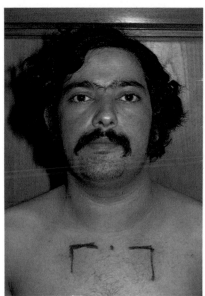

559

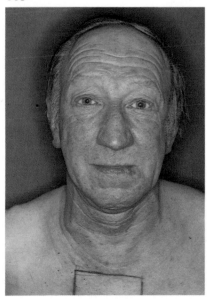

560 & 561 *Mediastinal obstruction* A later stage in the syndrome with glands pressing on the superior vena cava and producing obstruction of the neck veins but without facial plethora. A week later (**561**) there is increasing venous distension, fullness of the face, plethora, conjunctival injection and cyanosis.

562 *Mediastinal obstruction* This woman who had had a mastectomy for carcinoma presents the full blown picture of mediastinal obstruction. Note the plethora which extends from just below the breasts over the upper part of the body, cyanosis, oedema of the face, injection of the conjunctivae and dilated veins due to obstruction in the superior mediastinum of the great veins and on the trachea.

563 & 564 *Mediastinal obstruction* The final stage with dyspnoea, facial cyanosis and oedema – the eyes showing conjunctival injection. A common additional sign is dilated veins seen under the tongue due to back pressure from the obstruction (**564**).

560

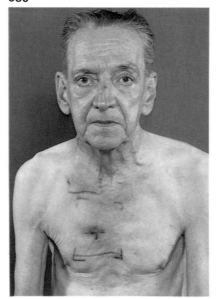

561

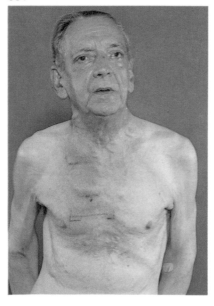

562

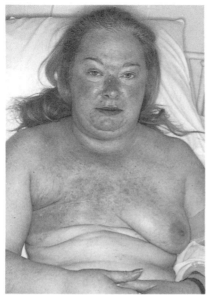

563

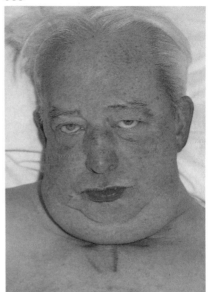

564

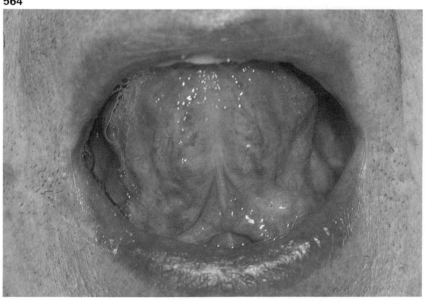

565 *Superior mediastinal obstruction* Dilation of the veins in the arms may also be seen in superior mediastinal obstruction and in very high elevations of the venous pressure. When tricuspid incompetence is present venous distension in the arm may have a pulsatile quality and may be used to find the level of the head of pressure by raising the arm above the right atrium.

566 *Elevated external jugular venous pressure* The upper limit on the column of blood can be seen in an old lady in congestive cardiac failure secondary to a high output state due to anaemia.

567 *Thickened nerves in the neck* The greater auricular nerve as it crosses the sterno-mastoid muscle may often be seen in leprosy and it should not be confused with dilated veins. The angle which the nerves make with the sterno-mastoid is different from the angle of the vein, apart from its consistency on palpation.

The cause here is leprosy: hypertrophy may also occur in other infiltrations with sarcoid tissue, neoplasms, reticuloses and amyloid. Other causes are hypertrophic polyneuropathies, following trauma and in neurofibromatosis.

568 *Distended neck veins, child* In a child distended neck veins are difficult to see and the easier indication of venous congestion is an enlarged liver.

565

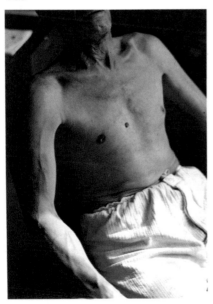

566

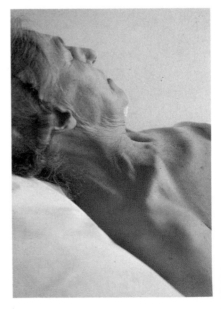

567

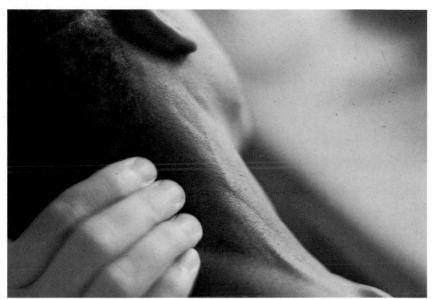

568

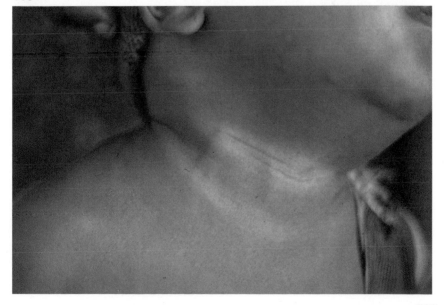

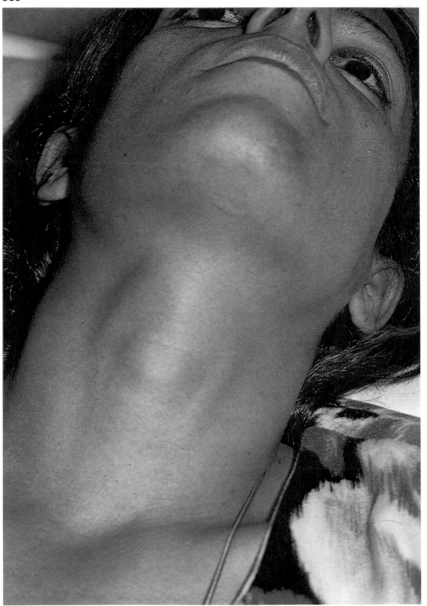

569 *Elevated internal jugular venous pressure* The head of the venous column is nearly to the angle of the jaw. When viewed with the trunk at 45° to the horizontal it was 10cm above the sternal angle (manubrio sternal junction). It is situated medial to the sterno-mastoid. The internal jugular vein is the best manometer for assessing venous pressure – it is straight and seldom kinks producing a false elevation.

A detailed analysis of the venous waves 'a', 'c', and 'v' presupposes an ability to note the elevated pressure in the first place. To do that one must know where to look and then differentiate the nerve, external jugular, internal jugular and arterial profiles by looking, palpating and timing the venous pulse and observing the effect of hepatic pressure on the venous column.

The prerequisites are: (1) a relaxed patient; (2) lying propped up at 45°; (3) a vein showing free oscillation with breathing and also with hepatic pressure and with the heartbeat; (4) differentiation from a fixed column due to proximal block.

570 & 571 *Right carotid aneurysm* No neurological defect. The sac can predispose to clot formation and subsequent emboli. Carotid pulsation in the neck may be due to: (1) aneurysm formation; (2) more commonly kinking of the right carotid artery often seen in females.

570

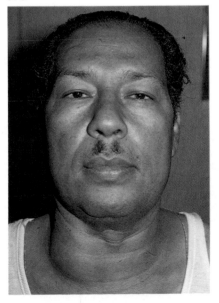

571

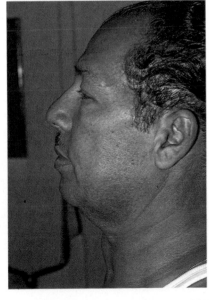

572 *Carotid body tumour* This is felt deeper than a branchial cyst posterior to the sternum mastoid and in its second two-thirds: it is solid, it does not vary in size, is not necessarily pulsatile and there may be a murmur. It does not move in a vertical plane though will move in a horizontal one.

573 *Carotid body tumour* Arteriogram.

Lymph gland enlargement in the neck

574 *TB lymphadenitis* Enlargement of the lymph gland in the upper cervical chain has to be distinguished from swellings about the ear such as sebaceous cysts, carotid tumours etc. The lymph gland enlargement is easily seen at the upper border of the sterno-mastoid.

575 *Hodgkin's disease* Bilateral lymph node enlargement in the upper cervical chain and tonsillar areas in a patient with Hodgkin's disease. *(Thomas Hodgkin, 1798–1866, described 1832).*

576 *Branchial cyst* The branchial cyst occurs further down the sterno-mastoid, peeps out of the middle third and may be partially covered by the muscle.

572

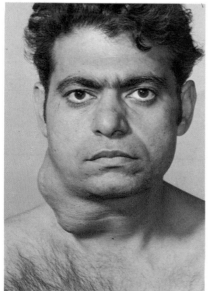

573

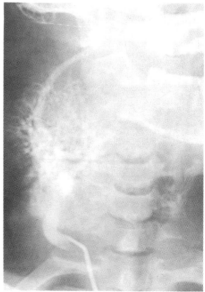

574

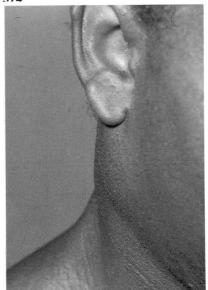

575

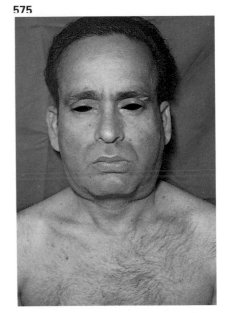

576

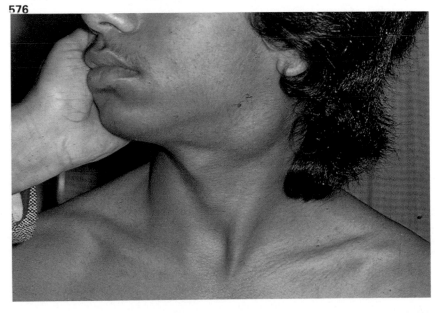

577 *Tuberculous lymph nodes in the neck* Incipient ulceration and sinus formation is typical of tuberculosis.

578 & 579 *Tuberculosis in the neck* Tuberculous lymphadenitis in a less acute stage when puckering of the skin takes place and sinuses form. The sinus in the midline communicates with the lesion in the supraclavicular fossa and pressure in the supraclavicular fossa produces an extrusion of caseous material from the midline (**579**).

Frequently TB in the neck has a superficial collection which communicates through the fascia with a deep collection – the collar stud abscess.

577

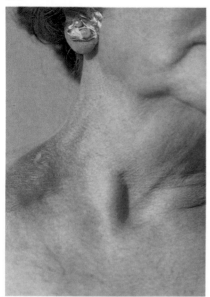

578

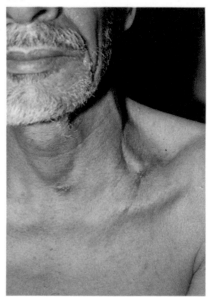

579

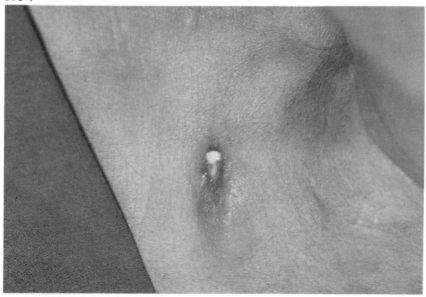

313

Radiology of the neck

The postgraduate student sometimes fails to appreciate the normal anatomy of the neck on the x-ray. This failure of appreciation leads to undue difficulty in interpreting findings in the neck and the next three x-rays are shown solely to bring out the simple anatomy in commonly viewed projections of the neck.

580 & 581 *Oblique view of the cervical spine* Anterior to the spine can be seen an air shadow of the trachea, anterior to this is shadow of the thyroid. It is important to appreciate the normal anatomy in the neck on radiology in order to interpret the significance of various swellings. This oblique view shows the intervertebral foramina. Do you know what these symmetrically disposed opacities are (*arrow*)? These should be regularly spaced counting down from the first cervical vertebra, but there is a gap between the third and fourth and then fourth and fifth, fifth and sixth, sixth and seventh are symmetrical again. This suggests that something has eroded the pedicles on the other side. This is confirmed when one looks at the oblique view from the other side showing a large intervertebral foramen distended by a neuro-fibroma.

582 *Lateral view of the neck: retropharyngeal abscess* This can be deduced without having seen an x-ray like this before solely from an understanding of the normal radiological appearances.

The important points to appreciate are: (1) the posterior margin of the tongue; (3) the air lucency cast by the air of the pharynx; (4) the posterior pharyngeal wall; (5) the hyoid bone; (6) this air space is the pharynx; (7) the thyroid cartilage; (2) the horizontal line of a gas-over-liquid fluid level.

It follows that the fluid level here (2) should pour over into the air space (6) but is bounded by the posterior pharyngeal wall. Furthermore the normal curve of the cervical spine has been lost, therefore one can postulate that the condition is painful with fluid lying posterior to the pharyngeal wall. It must be an abscess, retropharyngeal in site.

580

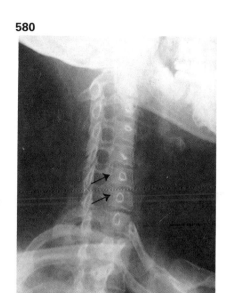

581

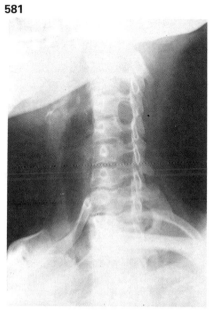

582

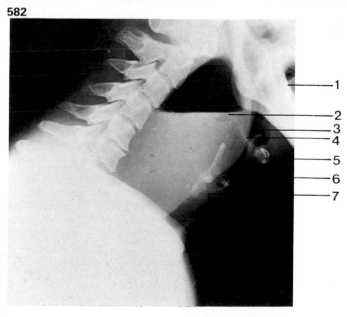

1

2
3
4

5

6

7

The Chest

EXAMINATION OF THE CHEST

The chest is examined by inspection, palpation, percussion, and auscultation. Some underlying facts are important and what follows contains my personal foibles. To 'examine the chest' means:

Inspection. The *nails* for clubbing, pallor or cyanosis. The *mucous membranes* for pallor or cyanosis. The *breasts* for gynaecomastia or asymmetry. The *chest* for shape (barrel chested = emphysematous, asymmetry = pulmonary fibrosis).

Palpation.
(1) Supra clavicular fossae – cervical rib, lymph gland.
(2) Equality of expansion. The careful assessment of expansion over the upper and lower chest can alert you to the presence of physical signs and is perhaps the best pointer to an underlying abnormality to be searched for by percussion and auscultation. The value of vocal tactile fremitus, particularly in assessing the presence and progress of a pleural effusion is often forgotten as it is sometimes easier to compare the vibrations felt by the hand and detect impairment which will help in assessment of reductions in percussion note over small collections of pleural fluid.
(3) Muscle bulk. Particularly the muscles of the shoulder girdle where wasting is easily noted.
(4) Movement and mediastinal shift. Presence of an abnormality in one side of the chest will impair the expansion of that side. A change in the volume of one pleural cavity over the other will result in a shift in the mediastinum towards the smaller volume. The zone – upper or lower – affected will determine whether the trachea or apex beats shift most. The value of minor variations in tracheal shift is dubious – a lot of time is wasted trying to detect minor variations. If good technique is adopted in the first place and the shift is not obvious, ignore it. If expansion is impaired look carefully for the shift.

Percussion. Compare side with side at the same level and in the same manner. The quality of the note will depend on the resounding properties of the thorax beneath – water, dull; air, very resonant. Between the two there are all gradations which will reflect the degree of 'airlessness' of the chest itself. Minor variations over a pleural effusion are often best appreciated by tactile vocal fremitus when the vibration is generated by the larynx as opposed to the vibration generated by the finger tip.

Auscultation. The value of auscultation depends on the conscious analysis of what is heard. Comparison of the two sides of the chest is paramount. The breath sounds are generated in the larynx and larger air passages. They are transmitted along the columns of air in the bronchi and through the air-containing lung to the chest wall, where they are picked up by the stethoscope. Changes in breath sounds are all related to physical change in the media through which the sound generated in the larynx and larger air passages has to pass. Solid lung produces excellent transmission if the bronchi are patent as the sound is not dissemminated but conducted to the chest wall in the same manner that the sound is conducted from the chest wall to the ear. If FLUID is placed between the lung and chest wall, the sound will be blocked at the lung/fluid interspace in the same way that sound is blocked if the ear is full of water after swimming; if air is placed in the pleural cavity the effect on the breath sounds is the same as placing the stethoscope 1 mm off the chest wall and listening for breath sounds.

Added sounds are dependent on patent bronchi and are produced on a reed vibration principle.

If the pleural cavity contains: (1) *Air* – breath sounds diminish, (2) *Fluid* – breath sounds diminish, (3) *Solid lung with patent bronchus* – breath sounds increase, (4) *Partial blocked bronchus* – breath sounds diminish, (5) *Crepitations* – a deep breath and a good cough will clear a majority of non pathological crepitations. The presence of post coughing (post tussive) crepitations is a cardinal physical sign; the presence of a post tussive rhonchus is a cardinal physical sign – both may indicate a physical change.

583 & 584 *The barrel chest* The ribs are lifted up to the horizontal in a fixed inspiratory position associated with emphysema. Breathing is diaphragmatic and expansion poor. The area of cardiac dullness and hepatic dullness may be smaller as the voluminous lungs cover the heart and liver and increase the resonance of percussion.

585 *Rickets (vitamin D deficiency)* The classic rosary. The bulges seen on the chest wall at the site of the costo-chondral junctions are produced by the expanded uncalcified matrix. Compare the photograph of the child's wrist (**460**), the pathology is the same.

Causes of rickets are: (1) dietary; (2) malabsorption; (3) renal failure; (4) renal tubular defects.

583

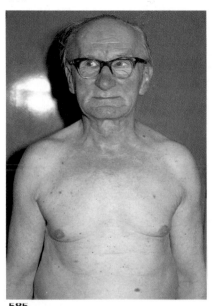

584

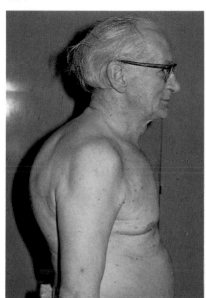

585

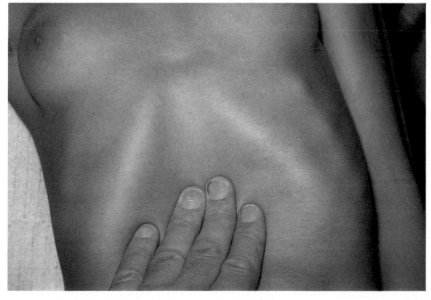

586 & 587 *Harrison's sulcus* The groove running laterally and slightly downwards, allegedly along the line of diaphragmatic attachment, where the pull of the diaphragm might pull in the rib.

The causes are: (1) congenital anomaly; (2) as a residue of rickets; (3) as a residue of asthma; (4) as a residue of chronic chest infection in childhood.

It may be combined with other abnormalities as in this case (lateral view), a mild degree of pectus excavatum (the depression at the lower end of the sternum). This abnormality may give an apparent increase in cardiac diameter on chest x-ray which can be discounted when the narrow AP diameter is noted on the lateral view. *(Edwin Harrison, 1779–1847, physician St Marylebone Infirmary, London.)*

588 *Chronic asthma* The development of the pectoralis muscles and the prominent sternum produce an early 'pigeon' chest.

589 *The acute asthmatic attack* The child fixes the shoulder girdle by supporting the arms on the couch and then uses his pectoralis major and sterno mastoid muscles as accessory muscles of respiration: hence their overdevelopment and the production of the characteristic chest. Note the flaring of the anterior nares which are also being used as accessory muscles of respiration.

586

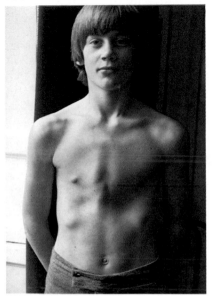

587

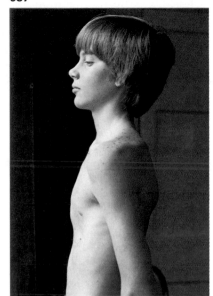

588

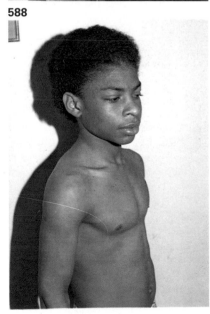

589

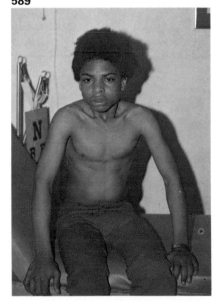

Pulmonary fibrosis

Clinically, note the flattening and the inequality of expansion of the chest. This is best noted by asking the patient to take a deep breath while standing some distance away at the end of the bed.

Scoliosis of the spine will throw part of the chest into prominence and the anterior part on the side of the convexity of the scoliosis will appear flattened. If no scoliosis exists the presence of flattening may indicate chronic unilateral pulmonary disease. The cause of the flattening is more often long standing fibrosis than pulmonary collapse. Flattening is usually associated with mediastinal shift.

590 & 591 *Ankylosing spondylitis* Costal expansion is negligible because of the loss of costo-vertebral movement caused by ankylosis. The kyphosis is fixed and the man's posture is a rigid one with no movement at all.

Consequently: (1) the prominent abdomen is not all fat but related to the need for diaphragmatic respiration; (2) the kyphosis is aggravated by his occupation as a hairdresser; (3) the x-ray shows calcification in the anterior spinal ligament and hyperextension between the skull and the atlas to keep the visual axis horizontal.

592 *Left upper lobe pulmonary fibrosis* Secondary to irradiation for left sided carcinoma of the breast. Note: (1) no left breast shadow; (2) trachea deviated to the left; (3) rib crowding in the left upper zone; (4) left hilum pulled upwards.

593 *Scarring due to repeated induction of an artificial pneumothorax* This is a clinical clue to tuberculosis in the past in a patient who presented with Addison's disease.

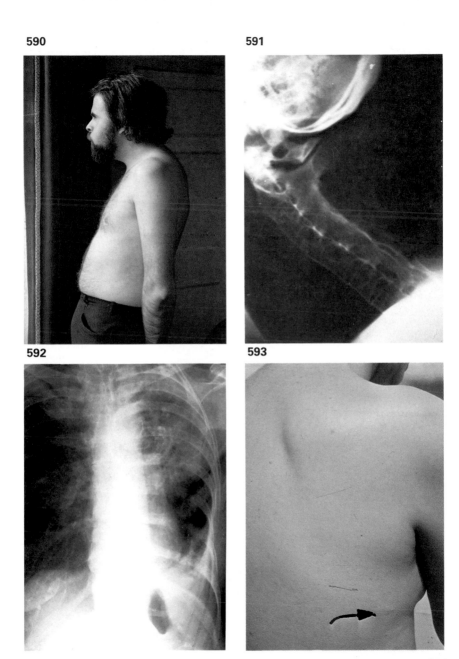

594–596 *Pott's disease* The chest deformity secondary to the gibbus of the spine reduces the vital capacity, an upset such as pneumonia or emphysema will then precipitate cardio respiratory insufficiency. The acute angulation due to vertebral destruction by tuberculosis can be seen in the x-ray. *(Sir Percivall Pott, 1714–1788, described 1779.)*

597 & 598 *Thoracoplasty* Posterior view shows relatively little deformity of the outline of the chest. When viewed from the front the change in the right axilla is easily seen.

594

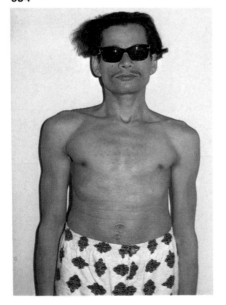

595

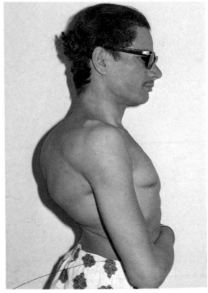

596

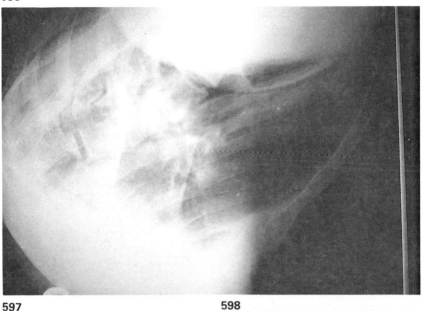

597

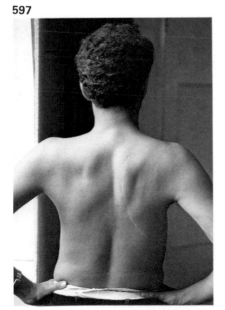

598

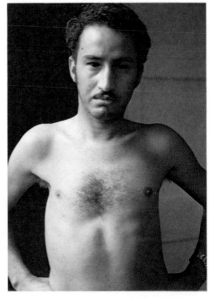

599 & 600 *Wasting* Recent weight loss is often easily appreciated in the skin of the upper chest and arms. It is lax, easily lifted and falls in folds.

601 *Winging of the scapula* Wasting and weakness of the muscles of the shoulder girdle may be first appreciated when examining the back of the chest. Winging of the scapula may be noted and wasting of the supra and infra spinatus is easily seen. Paralysis of serratus anterior (C567) is a not infrequent isolated finding, usually due to old polio or neuralgic amyotrophy.

602 *Campbell de Morgan spots* A capillary malformation of no significance – they do not blanch on pressure. They should not be confused with the spider naevus which occurs over this distribution.

599

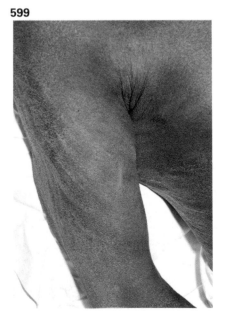

600

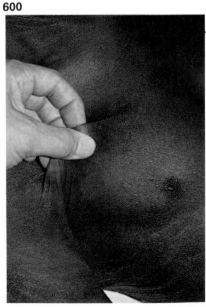

601

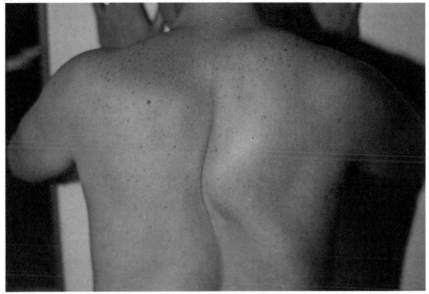

602

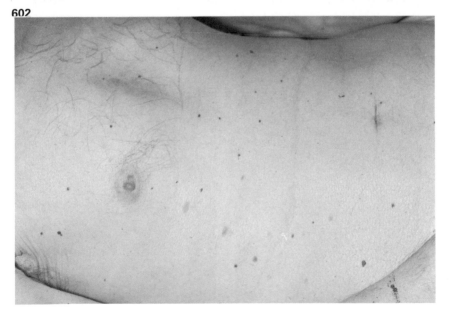

603 *Von Recklinghausen's disease (multiple neurofibromata)* This patient has an excess of brown café au lait spots. The normal individual can be expected to have between ten and twenty spots on the body. Once café au lait spots are noticed the other manifestations of multiple neurofibromatosis must be searched for: (1) neurofibromata (**604**); (2) pseudoarthrosis and orthopaedic abnormalities (**606** and **607**); (3) secondary effects of neurofibromata – acoustic neuroma, spinal tumour, neuropathic joint, rib notching; (4) associated conditions – phaechromocytoma, medullary carcinoma of the thyroid, glioma, medulloblastoma, lung cysts (honeycomb lung). *(Friedrich Daniel von Recklinghausen, 1833–1910, described 1882.)*

604 *Von Recklinghausen's disease* Multiple neurofibromata are present on the skin. The left arm is the site of a very large liponeurofibroma.

605 *Neuropathic knee joint (von Recklinghausen's disease)* Secondary to neurofibromata of the lumbar neural exit foramina.

606 *Von Recklinghausen's disease* In addition to the café au lait spots and cutaneous neurofibromata, this man has a pseudoarthrosis due to a bone lesion and a large neurofibroma of the left arm.

607 *Pseudoarthrosis in von Recklinghausen's disease, x-ray*

603   **604**

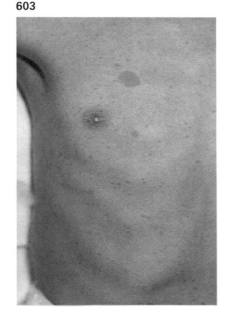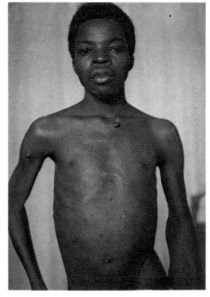

605

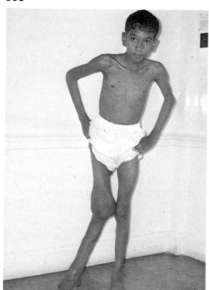

606

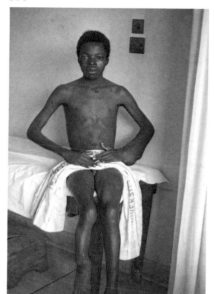

607

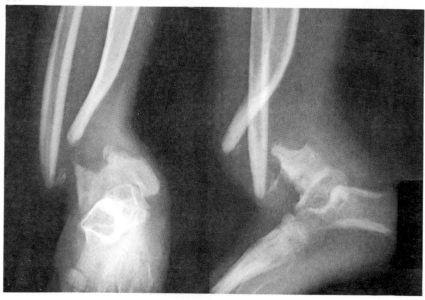

THE BREAST

608 *An accessory nipple* These may be seen anywhere along the milk line and in the female may enlarge at the time of menstruation and pregnancy.

609 *Absent left nipple* The scar of mastectomy in the male for carcinoma. It is important to appreciate the scar's significance as it may be relevant to the presenting complaint.

610 *Acute mastitis in the neonate* The active neonatal breast under the influence of maternal hormones is prone to manipulation by well meaning family. This may lead to a full blown mastitis as in this Nigerian infant. A similar mechanism accounts for neonatal menstruation.

611 *Neonatal menstruation* The uterine lining is sensitised by the high level of maternal oestrogens, sheds with oestren withdrawal after birth after which menstruation ceases.

608

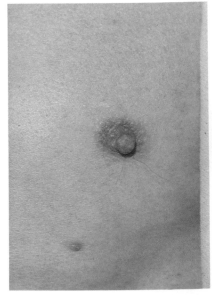

609

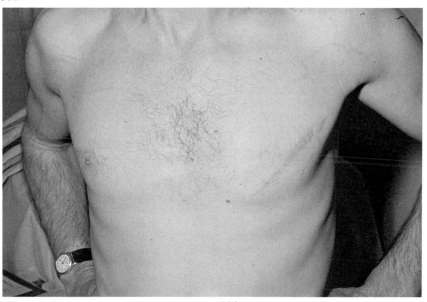

610

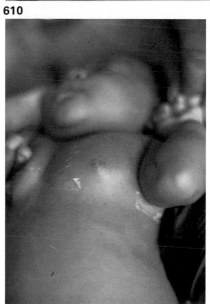

611

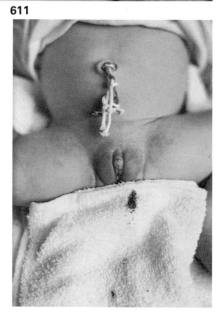

612 *Galactorrhoea* An acromegalic with hyperprolactinaemia: see **112–115**. Milking of the breast and squeezing of the nipple increases the flow. Galactorrhoea may be caused by: (1) drugs – phenothiazines, oral contraceptives, reserpine, tricyclic antidepressants; (2) pituitary tumours; (3) hypothalmic disease; (4) 'ectopic' prolactin production – lung tumours; (5) primary hypothyroidism; (6) chest wall injury – trauma, surgery, herpes zoster, by afferent reflex stimulation.

The mammary tissue develops under the influence of oestrogens – this produces the pubescent breast. Circulating prolactin induces nipple and areolar development and later secretion.

613 *The pituitary fossa of the preceding patient and a normal control, below*

614 *Gynaecomastia* A cirrhotic patient: spider naevii are present on the arm. Gynaecomastia may be unilateral or bilateral and must be differentiated from the pseudo gynaecomastia of obesity and tumours where there is no true increase in mammary tissue.

Causes: (1) at puberty; (2) re-feeding, after starvation or recovery from severe illness – probably due to resumed secretion of pituitary gonadotrophins suppressed during illness; (3) hypogonadism – primary testicular failure, Klinefelter's syndrome; (4) testicular tumours; (5) exogenous oestrogens; (6) liver disease; (7) drugs – spirolactone, isoniazid, reserpine and others; (8) other endocrine disorders – hyperthyroidism, diabetes; (9) non endocrine tumours; (10) pituitary tumours.

612

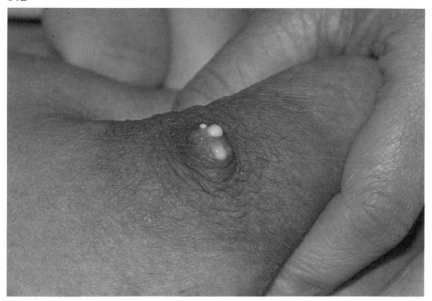

613

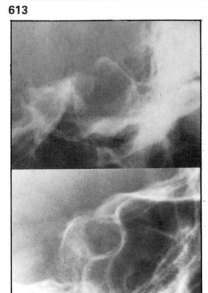

614

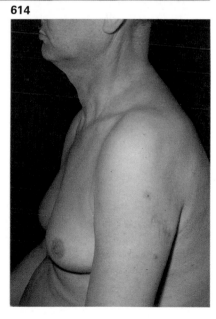

615 *Unilateral gynaecomastia* Gynaecomastia occurs physiologically at puberty with the surge of pituitary gonadotrophic hormones. In the male this is self limiting. An increase in size will also occur during pregnancy and lactation and under the stimulus of high prolactin levels in acromegaly.

616 *Klinefelter's syndrome (seminiferous tubule dysgenesis)* Breast enlargement secondary to hypogonadism.
   Other features are: often low normal intelligence; small firm 'pea sized' testes; small penis; poorly developed secondary sexual characteristics. *(Harry Fitch Klinefelter Jr., born 1912, described 1942.)*

617 *Gross weight loss with emaciation* An example of the weight loss of inadequate intake in an old man – yet the eyes are bright and he looks quite different from the cachexia of malignant disease in **629**.

615

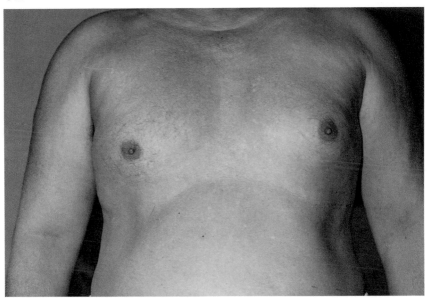

616

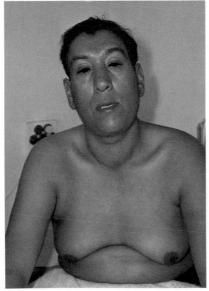

617

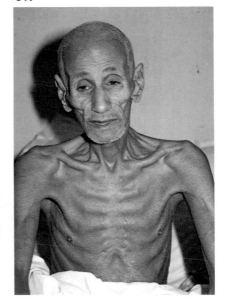

Once the anterior chest has been examined the patient is usually leant forwards and the back of the chest examined in the same way. At the same time check the sacrum and the loins.

618 *Bed sores* The result of neglect in a wasted patient who lay on his back – the ribs stick out and lead to pressure sores. Note the points on which the pressure occurs. Always check these areas, the sacrum, trochanters, medial condyles, femurs, heels and malleoli in any debilitated patient – particularly if the ward is understaffed. The earliest signs of redness may then be picked up before the skin breaks.

619 *The sacral pad of oedema* When the back is examined an opportunity exists for checking for pitting oedema over the sacrum. When a patient is first seen in out-patients or the consulting room he has been mobile and erect – once admitted to hospital and put to bed for 24 hours the ankle oedema may disappear only to appear, *if you look for it,* at the sacrum where the progress of getting rid of the excess fluid can be monitored.

620 *Spina bifida occulta* The tuft of hair over a spina bifida may be a clue in patients with neurological signs in the legs or difficulty with the bladder indicating neurological involvement.

618

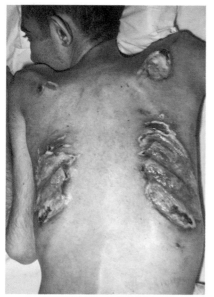

619

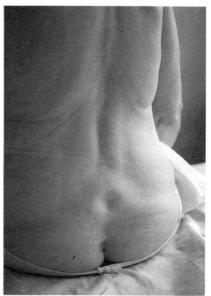

620

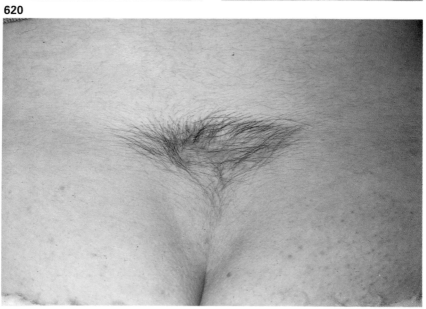

621 *Pilonidal sinus* The pouting granulation tissue at the opening of the sinus and the hairy natal cleft are usually present.

622 *Psoriasis* This may also be noted over the sacrum. It may be the only place where it is active at the time the patient is examined.

623 *Perinephric abscess* The filling of the loin and bulge with overlying redness. A diabetic presenting in precoma.

621

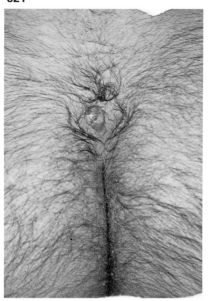

622

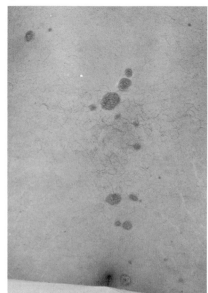

623

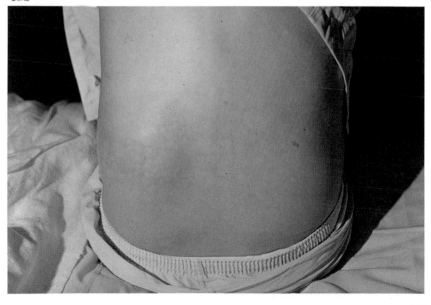

The Abdomen

EXAMINATION OF THE ABDOMEN

The posture of the hand

The most sensitive part of the hand is the fingerprint area: if all four are kept close together the sensation picture becomes of finer grain with no sensory gap between fingers, where anything might be happening (**624**).

The hand and forearm should remain straight (**625**), once the wrist flexes the finger tips themselves are being used and less information gained. It is useful to use the finger tips only if 'dipping' through fluid to bounce a viscus back at one's hand and identify its presence. The elbow and hand should be held at a tangent to the abdominal wall, though this may mean kneeling on the floor, to ensure that the palmar surface of the fingers is used. Think and feel, building up a mental picture to answer the questions: what is the site? size? shape? mobility? edge? resonance and tenderness? so that you do not need to palpate again.

Special points on palpation

The Liver. Probably the easiest viscus for the novice to feel but, if it is soft rather than firm, unless the edge flicks across the fingers one cannot be sure that it is enlarged though one may suspect it. Always begin well down in the right iliac fossa to ensure that the liver edge is caught as one moves up – the evidence comes with feeling the liver edge hit the radial edge of the finger tips. Naturally with a big firm liver there is little difficulty but attention to this detail will ensure that the liver is felt. Don't assume all swellings in the right upper quadrant are liver. The suprarenal mass can swivel down and be a differential diagnosis.

624

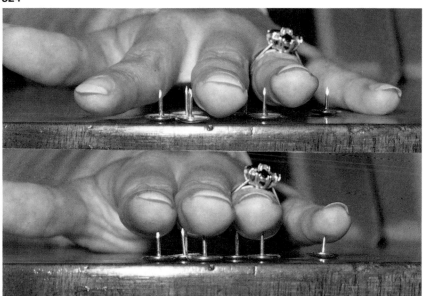

625

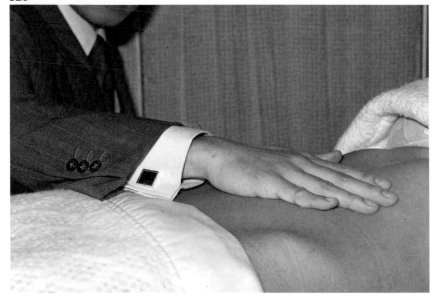

The Spleen (626). The enlarged spleen peeps out from under the left costal margin at a point between the mid clavicular and the anterior axillary line. A deep breath will sweep the spleen tip down the diaphragmatic dome to peep at the costal edge. The fingers (**627**) should form a continuation of the ribs so that the spleen follows down the fingers and is 'tipped'. If one pushes too hard a soft spleen will be missed, or the 11th rib, or the edge of the external oblique as it contracts, will be mistaken for the spleen. Light pressure will make tenderness more meaningful. The other hand is used to steady the ribs (see **627**). Many other manoeuvres have been suggested to bring out a spleen – lying the patient on his side etc.

Two additional points to remember are: ensure very good diaphragmatic movement, which means teaching the patient how to take a really deep diaphragmatic breath (without inducing tetany by hyperventilation). This is not always easy as it is the last 100ml intake of breath that will bring down the slightly enlarged spleen. The second is to percuss the costal margin if you *think* you feel the spleen; dullness on the costal margin that comes and goes with respiration is an additional piece of evidence. Finally if the spleen is not there just confirm that it is not *very* big and extending across the abdomen by feeling from the right iliac fossa across to the left costal margin – a very big spleen may be mistaken for a kidney.

Remember that a spleen: (1) peeps from the left costal margin; (2) you cannot get above it; (3) is dull to percussion; (4) has a notched medial edge.

626

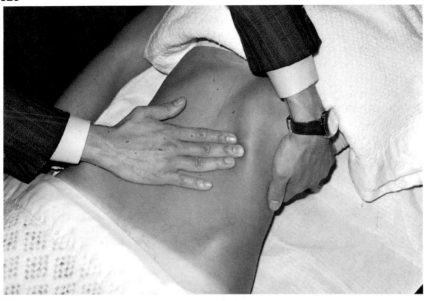

627

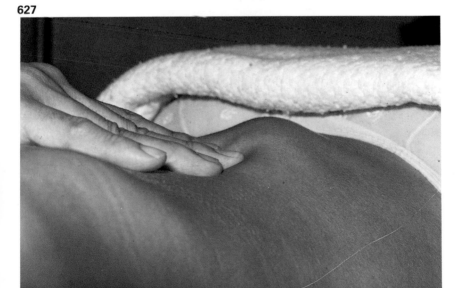

The Kidney. A common mistake is not to palpate bi-manually when routinely examining the abdomen. Probably the most difficult viscus to feel when minimally enlarged and even more difficult to decide on the borderline between normal and abnormal. The kidney moves with respiration. The lower poles may be palpable under normal circumstances in the thin individual with a good diaphragmatic excursion. The essence of examination (**628**) is the sensation felt by the left hand, the hand placed in the loin which enables one to feel the kidney *bi-manually.* It follows that the hands must be pressed together closely enough to be only the kidney's thickness apart and firmly enough to press the kidney onto the loin hand – to do this requires relaxation on the part of the patient. Often the patient will relax better if you can get him to talk and the right hand (anterior) must burrow into the belly with each breath going nearer to apposition of the two hands with each inspiration.

628

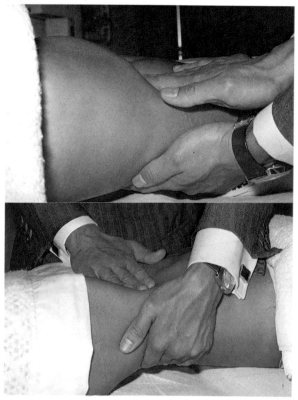

The procedure in examining the abdomen

Look at the legs. Is there oedema? (may be very relevant to cirrhosis and pelvic tumours).

Look at the hands. Is there palmar erythema or a contracture? Are the nails white, brown?

Look at the skin. Are there stigmata of liver disease, jaundice, stretch marks, spiders?

Feel the supraclavicular fossae. Are there any glands? (The lymphatic drainage of the stomach goes up on the left to the supraclavicular fossa.)

Look at the umbilicus. Check for eversion, hernia and lumps.
Look at the hernial orifices.
Look at the shadows on the abdomen. Using an oblique light watch the play of the shadows across the belly and the changes with respiration produced by masses moving behind the abdominal wall. A great deal will be seen, and often more will be seen than felt. Note the movement of the abdominal wall with respiration (it will be minimal with peritoneal irritation) : the changing shadows of visible peristalsis – a late sign of intestinal obstruction but a normal finding in those with a divarication of the recti or a thin abdominal wall. Note the contours of the belly: symmetry – fluid, flatus, foetus; asymmetry – an enlarged viscus or mass.

Palpation. If your hand is cold palpate initially through blankets. Always leave the area you think is painful to last because once pain has been felt the patient will anticipate further pain and will not relax adequately. Watch the patient's facial·expression for the earliest sign of pain – test rebound tenderness only when you finish the examination.

Percussion. Useful to find the liver edge (both upper and lower borders) and to check the spleen as well as the bladder, uterus etc. It's best to progress from resonant to dull. Initially percuss lightly.

Auscultation. This is only of value if practised regularly – you always feel the abdomen, why shouldn't you always listen to it: the silence will then be appreciated for what it means and the difference between normal sounds and hyper-active ones appreciated.

Listen for the following sounds: (1) femoral bruit, (2) hepatic bruit – hepatoma, (3) coeliac bruit – may be normal, or a pointer in ischaemic colitis, (4) renal bruit – in hypertension listen to the abdomen and in the renal angle, (5) the splash of the obstructed pylorus.

The swollen belly

Fluid in the peritoneal cavity (ascites). The features are: the general distension and umbilical eversion; the feel of a 'hot water bottle'; shifting dullness (you must demonstrate dull flanks first to show a shift); fluid thrill – usually demonstrates the obvious in ascites but will prove that a lump is a fluid-containing cyst.

Diagrammatically ascites is:

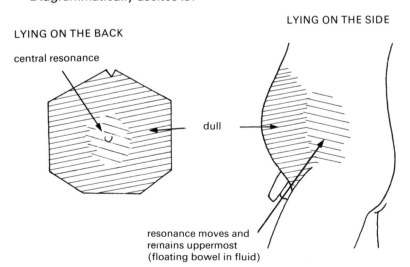

LYING ON THE SIDE

LYING ON THE BACK

central resonance

dull

resonance moves and remains uppermost (floating bowel in fluid)

General gut distension. The features are: distended belly; generalised resonance.

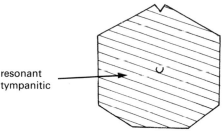

resonant
tympanitic

Ovarian cyst/pregnancy and fibroid/big bladder. These three all show similar physical signs. Differentiate on the history initially.

Percussion will demonstrate the mass arising from the pelvis. (1) Does not move with respiration, (2) can't get below it, (3) dull to percussion, (4) confirm rectally and vaginally, (5) does it move the cervix?

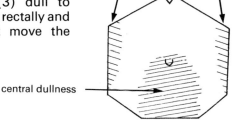

resonant flanks

central dullness

Masses that move with respiration

These must be moved either by the diaphragm or by a viscus which is moved by the diaphragm.

The liver. Features: it extends from the right costal margin to the left costal margin; it enlarges downwards to the right iliac fossa; the edge is regular; it moves with respiration; the surface is smooth (but knobbly in cirrhosis and shows umbilicated nodules in secondary tumour); you can't get above it.

Note: do not be misled into diagnosing a big liver by feeling the edge of a Riedel's lobe laterally. *(Bernard Moritz Karl Ludwig Riedel, 1846–1916.)*

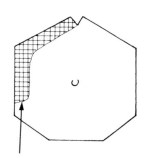

Riedel's lobe

The spleen. Feel in the right place on the costal margin with the correct technique. Percuss it if in doubt. Make the patient breathe with a big diaphragmatic excursion. Check you are not feeling the external oblique muscle or a floating rib tip.

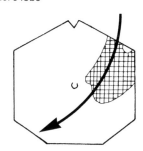

The kidney. You may feel the lower poles in the normal person. Feel the kidney with the hand in the loin bi-manually, be alert to the feeling in the loin hand. Listen for bruit front and back.

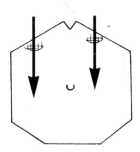

The gall bladder. Features: it's under the right costal margin, is ovoid, and moves with respiration.

Faeces. These will indent and will disappear with an enema.

Central abdominal masses

These may be: glands; a pancreatic cyst (it doesn't move); a mesenteric cyst (it moves diagonally as it is in the mesentery, *see diagram*); a central vertebral mass with the aorta overlying it, often felt by patients (the aorta is pulsatile, an aneurysm expansile). A mass in the epigastrium may be stomach, pancreas, glands or liver. A mass in the right iliac or left iliac fossae or in the periphery of the abdomen should always be checked after an enema, especially if it indents with pressure, it may be faeces.

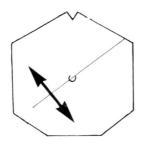

Differential diagnosis

Big spleen. This has a notch in the medial edge and extends from the left costal margin to the right iliac fossa.

Big liver. It has a characteristic edge, you can't get above it.

Big kidney. Felt bi-manually. (1) the loin hand feels it move with respiration and the anterior hand presses the kidney onto it – the reverse movement of squeezing a bar of wet soap out of cupped hands. (2) it's resonant: the colon passes over it.

Big lump. Differentiate the spleen, liver and kidney from each other to decide on the origin of the big lump and thereby which system is involved. This may be much more difficult than determining the underlying pathology. After you decide which viscus is responsible for or related to the lump *then* you can decide which investigation to order first.

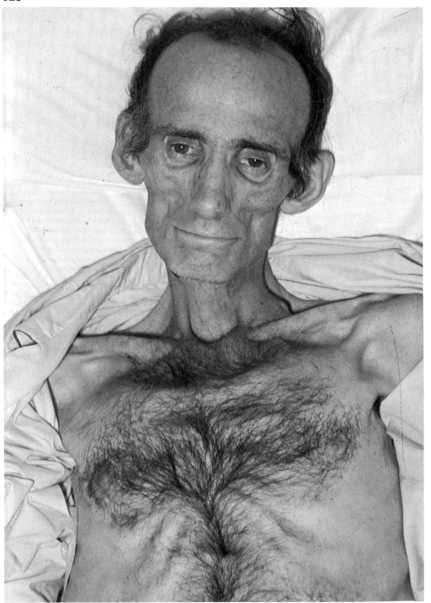

629 *Troisier's sign* Enlargement of the gland in the left supraclavicular fossa in a patient with carcinoma of the stomach. Drainage occurs straight upwards and the left supraclavicular fossa should always be palpated when carcinoma of the stomach is suspected, even though no mass is felt in the stomach. *(Charles Emile Troisier, 1849–1919.)*

630 & 631 *Ovarian cyst* The presenting complaint was a puffy right leg; minimal swelling of the leg may be due to pressure on lymphatics and veins by a pelvic mass which is not easily felt per abdomen.

This young Cypriot girl, a dressmaking machinist, complained of heaviness in the leg at the end of the day. She adjusted the pace of her sewing machine by pressure from the right foot onto a treadle. No local cause was found, the abdomen was normal on palpation, rectal examination unremarkable and she had no haemoglobinopathy – her only other symptom was occasional difficulty with micturition. The IVP showed up the pelvic mass, later confirmed on vaginal examination. The moral is embarrassingly obvious.

630

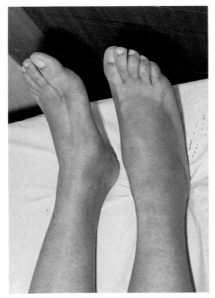

631

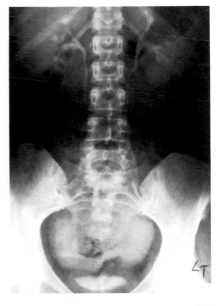

632 *Striae distensiae* Affects the abdomen, buttocks, thighs, breasts and upper arms. Most frequently seen: in obesity; in pregnancy (striae gravidarum); in Cushing's syndrome; with systemic steroids and ACTH; with local application of steroids.

The colour sequence is white – pink – red – purple – white. In these conditions there is a change in the glucocorticoid status – the site and direction of the striae being related to the mechanical tensile stress imposed on the skin by the weight gain, in itself an important factor in addition to the suppression of fibroblastic activity and change in collagen behaviour. Histologically elastic fibres are absent in the centre of the lesion, and curled up at the edge. The dermis is thinned and collagen fibres separated.

633 *Cautery* This sort of sight on examining the abdomen should not lead to confusion – it indicates: (1) abdominal pain; (2) generalised; (3) probably pain of long standing; (4) it relaxes and remits – remission short lived; (5) the fact that you are being consulted shows it did not work and the patient has decided to put his trust in the Devil he does *not* know.

632

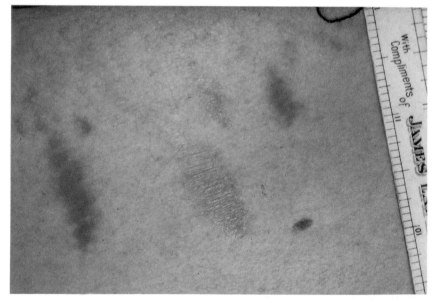

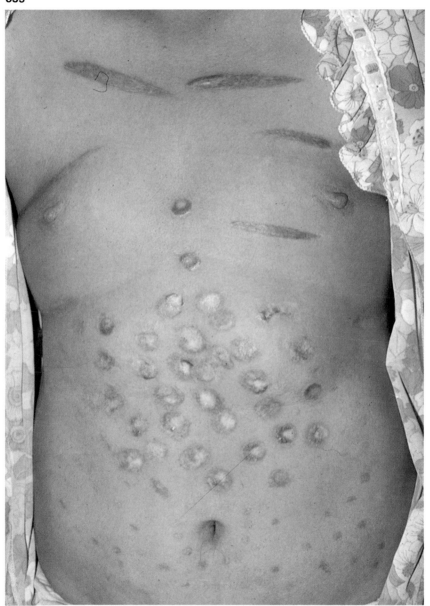

Examination of the umbilicus may produce an unexpected clue to the pathology. Acute inflammation, secondary deposits, discharges due to poor hygiene or congenital abnormalities, herniae and dilated venous systems may all be seen.

634 *Umbilical hernia* The normal umbilicus is inverted. Umbilical eversion is present – this may be due to: (1) hernia; (2) increase in abdominal content – fluid, flatus, viscera, tumour.

This hernia may be a congenital central weakness and occurs frequently in: the protein deficient African child; the obese, in whom perhaps a congenital weakness gives way; and ascites when a previously unnoticed hernia can be seen to fill with fluid on standing erect (**650**).

In this case a tuberculosis peritonitis with ascites was the cause of the abdominal fullness. The coiled worm under the skin is a guinea worm (dracunculus medinensis) which has got lost and calcified (see **738**).

635 *Umbilical sepsis* The cord has been cut with a portion of old razor blade and some mud and dung applied as an immediate dressing. Cellulitis of the abdominal wall is present. Note the 'peau d'orange' due to oedema pulling on the skin septa.

636 *Umbilical sepsis* This condition is common in West Africa where it is the practice to sever the cord with a piece of bamboo stick and possibly to rub in cow dung as a dressing. This leads to sepsis and is a frequent portal of entry for tetanus in the neonate.

637 & 638 *Secondary deposits at the umbilicus* (1) Carcinoma body of uterus. (2) Carcinoma ovary. Abdominal primaries may seep through the umbilicus and a secondary may be felt in the umbilicus. It is important to look and feel since the umbilical secondary deposit may be deep in the umbilical scar. In these two patients the umbilical sign was the presenting feature.

634

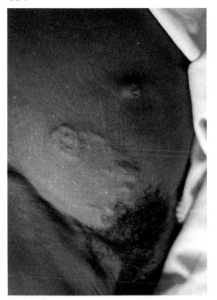

636

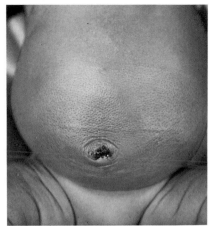

637

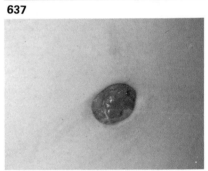

635

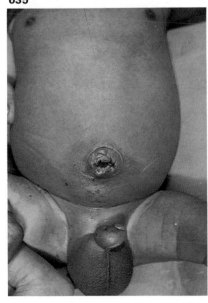

638

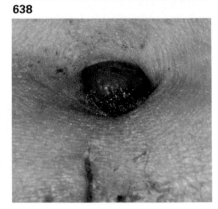

639

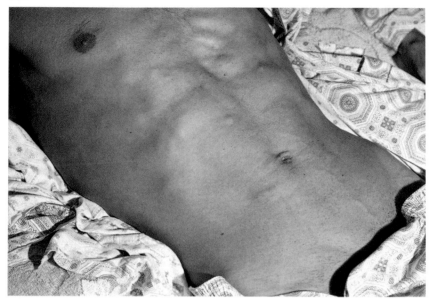

640

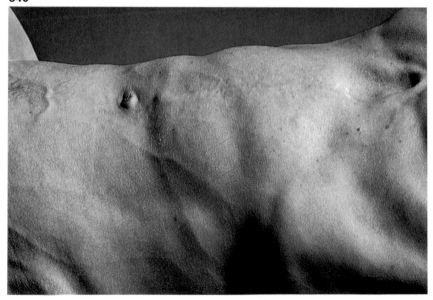

Dilated veins on the trunk may be due to: (1) vena caval block or compression; (2) portal hypertension; (3) portal vein thrombosis.

The consequences may be varices, splenomegaly, dilated surface veins (collaterals), intractable piles.

639 *Inferior vena caval obstruction (oblique lighting)* Dilated veins, whose flow is upwards, can be seen in the lower abdomen, and also in the mid-axillary line. A nodule in the liver, which moves when the patient breathes, can be seen to the right of the midline in the epigastrium.

640 *Carcinoma oesophagus and hepatic secondaries (oblique lighting)* An extensive venous collateral network is seen over the abdomen – flow is upwards to bypass the obstructed inferior vena cava. Note: the large liver whose edge can be seen just above the umbilicus and on either side of the midline.

641 *Para aortic metastases from carcinoma bladder leading to IVC compression and collateral venous systems* A particularly good example. Flow upwards.

641

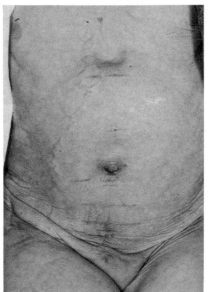

The swollen abdomen or fullness of the belly

This is usually associated with umbilical eversion (**634**). The abdomen has a particular look to it (**651**) if even a little fluid is present. The look is confirmed by the characteristic feel of a bag full of water as waves oscillate away from the point of touch and back from the edge again.

A swollen abdomen may be due to:

(1) big incisional herniae. ⎡ *All these will produce*
(2) gas, flatus. | *generalised swelling with*
(3) fluid.   ⎣ *specific physical signs.*
(4) viscera: liver, spleen, kidney, pancreas. Localised swelling and specific signs.
(5) tumour – anywhere, many signs.
(6) swellings arising out of the pelvis. Similar physical sign. Differentiate by specific direct questions: big bladder, big ovarian cyst, pregnant uterus.
(7) abdominal proptosis or hysterical bloating.

642 & 643 *Abdominal proptosis* A frequent cause of transient abdominal swelling and feeling of distension. It may come on rapidly and the patient is obliged to wear loose clothes. It is a little recognized and rarely sought physical sign. 'Now show me how it looks . . .' – the patient can often demonstrate the change in abdominal contour while being examined (produced by a combination of diaphragmatic descent and increased lumbar lordosis). It is nearly always a manifestation of 'stress': when chronic this is the mechanism of pseudocyesis.

642

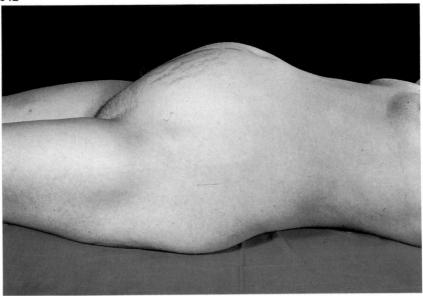

643

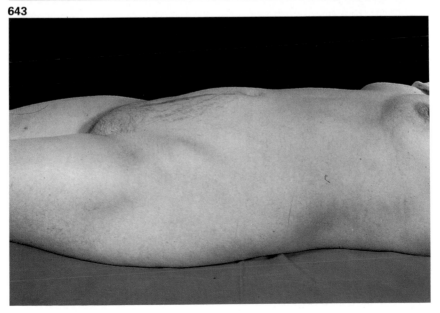

644 *Hernia* An incisional hernia in a patient with chronic bronchitis who had an operation for duodenal ulcer, the wound became infected and broke down.

645 *The scaphoid abdomen* The name given for the concavity of the abdomen seen in weight loss and in dehydration – sometimes in rigidity with no respiratory movement. A secondary deposit of growth in the liver can be seen in the midline which moves with respiration. A similar appearance is seen in an epigastric hernia through the linea alba but no movement will occur with respiration.

646 *Peritonitis* The tumescent abdomen in late-stage peritonitis has a characteristic shape which should be contrasted with the abdomen of ascites (**650**), and the scaphoid abdomen of weight loss or rigidity (**645**). This patient had carcinoma of the stomach and was operated upon. In the post operative period he insidiously developed peritonitis secondary to a ruptured anastomosis. The condition developed under the cover of analgesics.

644

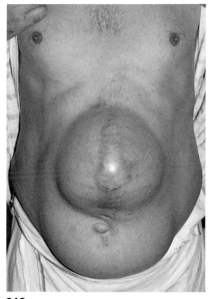

645

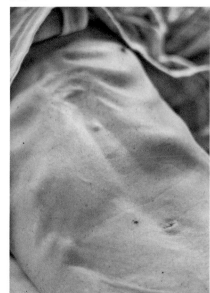

646

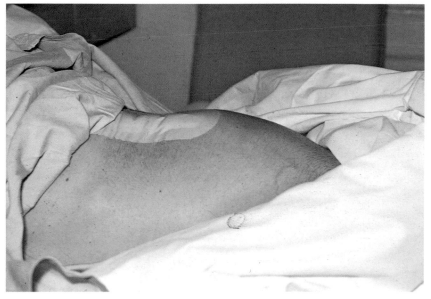

Ascites

A litre of fluid at least will be present before ascites can be detected clinically. The abdomen will be swollen, the swelling generalised, the umbilicus everted, the flanks dull to percussion, the centre resonant – if the flanks *are* dull then demonstrate shifting of dullness by turning the patient on the side and showing that a previously dull area is now resonant.

A fluid thrill will only occur with fluid under tension, it is present in ascites when the fluid is obvious and is then an additional sign only. Fat and fluid may both give a thrill to the inexperienced! A fluid thrill is of more use in demonstrating fluid in a tense mass.

647 *Tuberculosis of the peritoneum* Note the abdominal distension, everted umbilicus and glandular enlargement of the left groin. At first sight, the swelling in the left groin gives the appearance of a psoas abscess.

648 *Gross ascites* Note the total umbilical eversion – and wasting. A resonant central abdomen with gas filled gut floating at the top. Fluid thrill and shifting dullness present – gas filled gut floats to the top when the patient lies on the side, so the resonant area remains uppermost and the dullness has shifted position.

649 *Gross ascites (TB)* Emaciated. Peripheral oedema. Tense fluid filled belly. The swelling generalised over the abdomen. Look at the neck veins, check for pulsus paradoxus to exclude constrictive pericarditis.

650 *Cirrhosis of the liver* Note the jaundiced eye, the distended abdomen from ascites, the full umbilicus and gynaecomastia.

Other physical signs to look for are: jaundice, **37**; white nails, **45**; shiny nails, **655**; liver palms, **44**; liver feet, **796**; spiders, **41**; scratch marks, **658**; oedema, **649**; Troisier's sign, **629**; palpable gall bladder, **654**; gynaecomastia, **614**; distended veins, **639**.

647

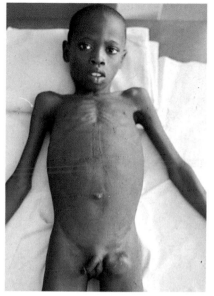

648

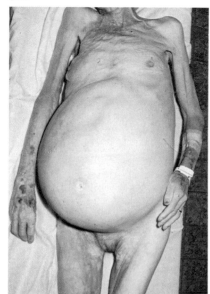

649

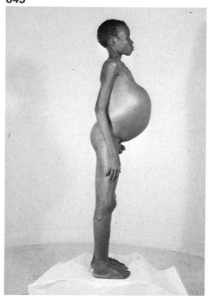

650

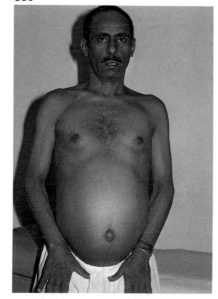

651 *Cirrhosis of the liver* Note the empty umbilicus now that the patient is lying flat (Cf. **650**), bilateral gynaecomastia and the distended abdomen (ascites).

652 *Haemochromatosis (hepatosplenomegaly)* Note the grey colour of the skin, the absent chest and axillary hair.

653 *Haemochromatosis (cirrhosis)* Observe: gynaecomastia, spider naevii, and a liver biopsy dressing. The clue is the sparse axillary hair — then check the genitals.

651

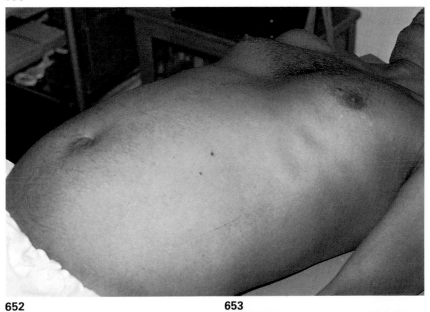

652

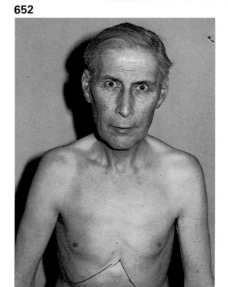

653

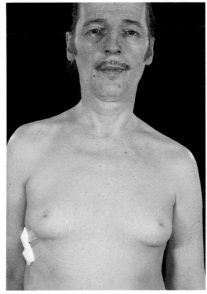

654 *The palpable gall bladder* It may be visible if viewed by oblique light. It moves with respiration and lies more laterally than usually taught – i.e. the lateral border of the rectus. It is easy to see how faulty selections of a site for liver biopsy – too far anterior – brings one perilously near to the gall bladder.

As a general rule if there is obstructive jaundice and a palpable gall bladder then the obstruction is of the common bile duct. A stone in the cystic duct and one in the common bile duct is the exception.

655 *Jaundice, carcinoma of pancreas* In jaundice look at the nails: if the tips have a mirror-like polish then he has intractable skin irritations and may have obstructive jaundice. Look for scratch marks – is the gall bladder felt?

656 & 657 *Itching, scabies* If the nails are polished and there is no jaundice don't forget to check the finger webs and wrist creases for the burrows of scabies. Remember that scabies spans all social classes.

Itching will produce: polished nails, excoriation, lichenification, pigmentation.

All these changes will modify the way the original rash/change looked. Grossly infected scabies does not look like **656** – so one's index of suspicion must be high.

654

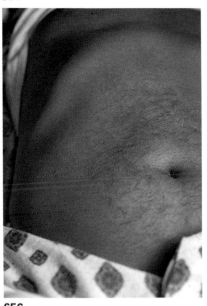

655

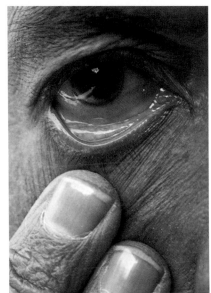

656

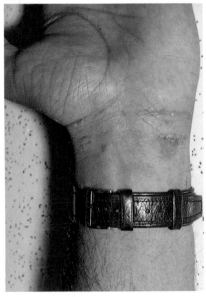

657

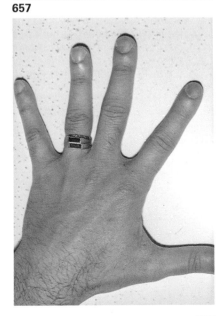

658 *Excoriation of the back induced by itching* This patient had early obstructive jaundice. Before the appearance of the jaundice he developed intense itching. Note that the marks are in a line produced by scratching with the left hand reaching round to the right side of the back. If did not occur in that part of the back which the patient cannot reach.

659 & 660 *Onchocerciasis (buttocks)* Parasitic infestation is a common cause of itching – the friction leads to secondary changes in the skin with lichenification or infection. This condition is due to infestation with onchocerciasis volvulus, a filarial worm common in West Africa but may be seen in visitors.

The worm encysts itself beneath the skin and gives rise to intense itching with lichenification and nodule formation of the skin. It is important that the pruritus is not misdiagnosed as scabies and that the vitiligo which occurs is not mistaken for leprosy. The onchocercial eye disease, or river blindness, may be confused with conjunctivitis and trachoma. The diagnosis is easy by lifting some skin with a needle and taking a snip and examining it under the microscope, as has been done here.

661 *Itching, Hodgkin's infiltrate* Itching may be symptomatic of a skin or systemic disease. The causes are: (1) *nerves,* neuro dermatitis; (2) *senile atrophy,* the itch of the aged may be intractable; (3) *parasites* – the louse on the skin, scabies into the skin, onchocerciasis under the skin; (4) *liver disease,* probably due to bile salts either in obstructive jaundice or preceding jaundice in chronic active hepatitis or as a symptom of primary biliary cirrhosis; (5) *malignancy,* carcinoma, infiltrating the skin (Hodgkin's disease, lymphoma); (6) *drug reaction;* (7) *eczema;* (8) *diabetes;* (9) *uraemia* – syphilitic rashes *usually* do not itch. *(Thomas Hodgkin, 1798–1866, described 1832.)*

658

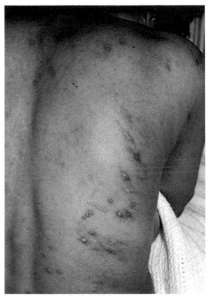

659

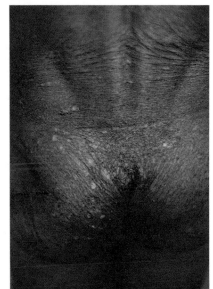

660

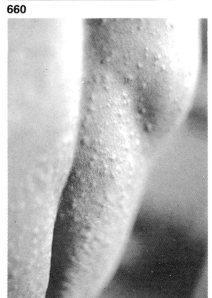

661

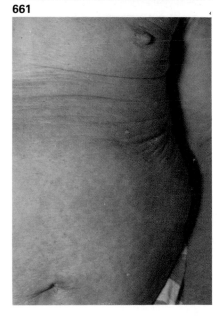

The anus and excreta

662 *The silver stool* The appearance of steatorrhoea together with mild blood loss, e.g. ampullary carcinoma.

663 *Steatorrhoea* Occult steatorrhoea may be a formed stool. The fat-laden stool is usually bulky, floating, offensive and difficult to flush. But the normal stool of high gas content will also float.

664 *Self-induced diarrhoea* Remember patients can tease! Self-induced diarrhoea diagnosed by adding caustic soda to the stool – surreptitious phenolthalein taking revealed.

665 & 666 *Fixed drug eruption* A clue to laxative addiction. This patient had an eruption which appeared whenever he took laxatives containing phenolthalein. This is a good example of the post inflammatory hyperpigmentation which may persist indefinitely. It may also occur with barbiturates and with sulphonamides. The characteristic of the fixed drug reaction is that the rash occurs at the same site on each exposure to the drug.

662

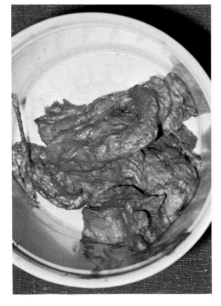

663

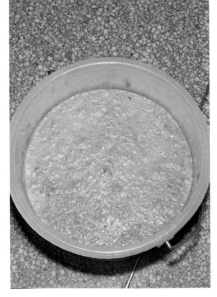

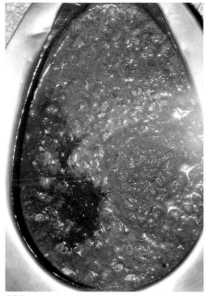

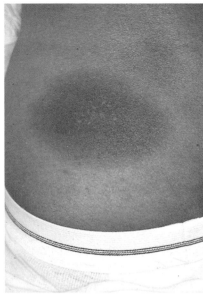

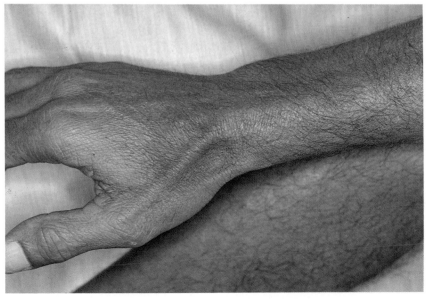

667 & 668 *Ulcerative colitis and the skin* The initial lesion is a red area (**667**). This develops into a sterile purulent blister (**668**). Compare the sequence of cancrum oris.

669 & 670 *Pyoderma* When severe and intractable to medical treatment (**669**) it may be an indication for colectomy – which allows rapid healing. Two weeks after colectomy, **670**.

667

668

669

670

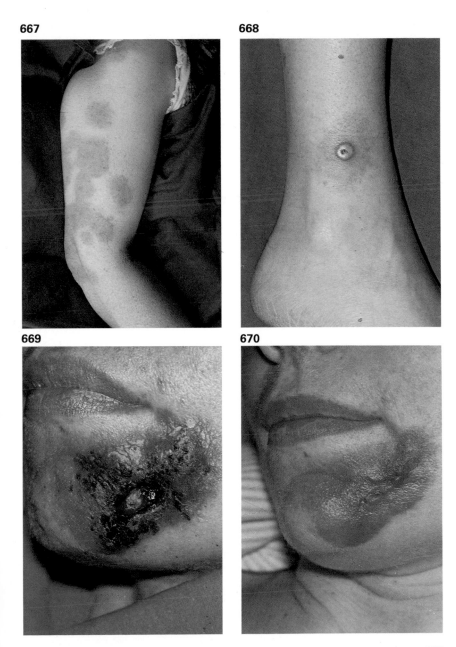

671 *Rectal prolapse in diarrhoea* A common finding in severe diarrhoea, especially in children. Manual replacement may be all that is necessary.

672 *Pruritus ani* The lichenified pink-white skin change is typical of chronic itch. The cause is usually long lost and remains a cycle of itch-scratch-itch. In children think of thread worms which lay their eggs at the anal verge and produce intractable irritation. Skin tags, the remnants of thrombosed external piles, are seen.

673 *Acute thrombosed external piles* A painful self-limiting condition.

671

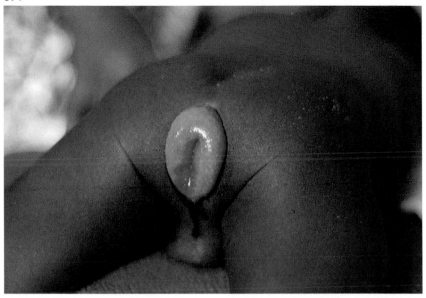

672

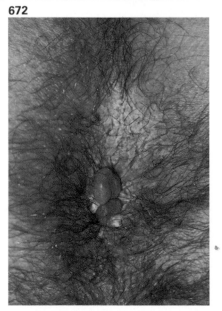

673

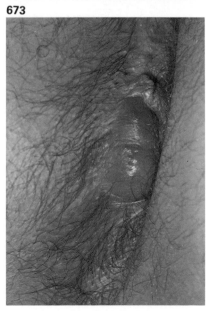

674 *Internal haemorrhoids* Seen up the proctoscope as the patient strains. With withdrawal the haemorrhoids prolapse and are captured by the anal sphincter. A common cause of rectal bleeding and insidious anaemia – they should never be automatically assumed to be the cause of the passage of blood.

675 *Acute anal fissure and sentinel pile* A very painful condition. Parting the skin folds will bring the apex of the fissure to view, even if digital examination is difficult. The sentinel pile is seen at the external edge, with the scarlet of the fissure deep to it.

676 *The anal fistula (Crohn's disease ≡ regional ileitis)* Twenty-five per cent of patients with intestinal Crohn's disease may have an anal lesion during their illness: it may be the presenting feature and may antedate the abdominal disease. Biopsy is important to differentiate other causes – TB, simple fistula, etc.

674

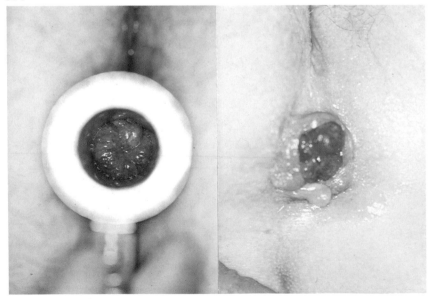

675

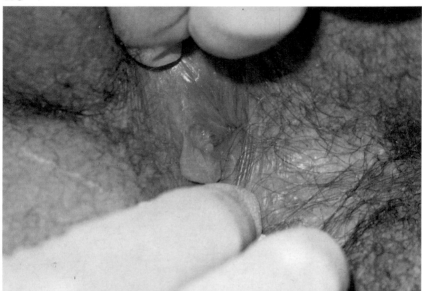

676

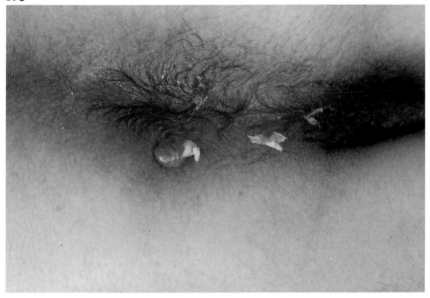

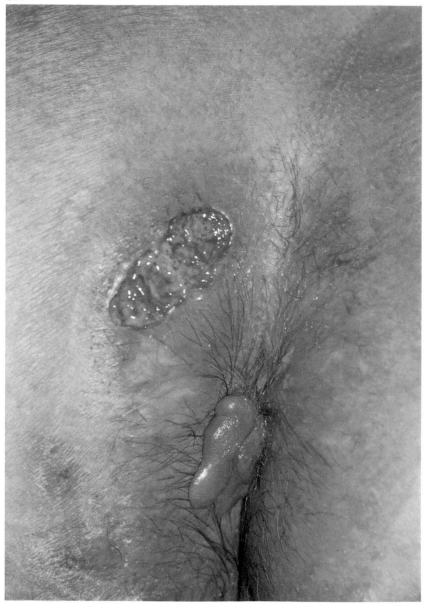

677 *The anal fistula and anal tags (Crohn's disease)* Many fistulae may be present – often surprisingly painless. The skin tags look succulent and soft but are of a very firm consistency; the dusky blue appearance is characteristic. Biopsy will show the characteristic histology. *(Burril Bernard Crohn, born 1884, described in 1932.)*

678 *Swollen testicle and sinus* Before completing abdominal examination – feel the testicles! Examination of the rectum and genitalia are two places where attention to clinical method pays dividends time and again.

This patient came to England to consult doctors. He came for a 'general check up'. At the end of the negative abdominal palpation, the genitalia were examined and a swelling with a sinus found (*arrow*). On remonstrating with the patient and pointing out his obvious abnormality he said that this was his reason for travelling to England and he wanted to see if the doctor found it as he would then feel that he was being properly examined and could place his care in the doctor's hands. The patient's method of quality control.

678

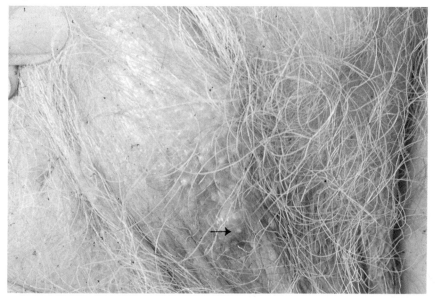

The Lower Limbs

679 *Obesity, adipose dimpling and oedema* No pitting. There may be oedema as a secondary effect due to the sheer physical weight obstructing the venous and lymphatic return as can be seen in the feet. This oedema will pit.

680–682 *Oedema* A pit can be produced on pressure by displacement of the extra-cellular fluid by the fingers. This pressure may need to be firm and sustained for thirty seconds to produce the characteristic pit.

This man had a venous thrombosis of the leg. Note the loss of bony landmarks, the shininess of the skin and the pressure mark produced by the supporting stockings on the foot. The finger is placed on the foot (**681**) and pressure is exerted for thirty seconds and released (**682**) leaving the characteristic pit which is caused by displacement of fluid and where even the fingerprint can be seen. The physical signs will be the same no matter what the cause of the oedema, be it inflammatory, hypoproteinaemic, due to cardiac failure or sodium retention, with the exception of congenital lymphoedema where the swelling may be 'brawny' and not pit so easily on pressure.

679

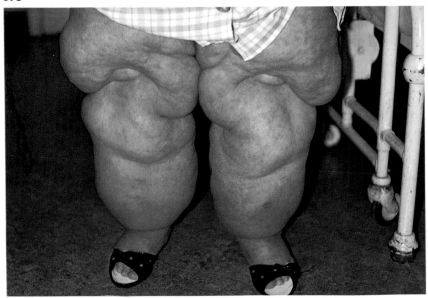

680

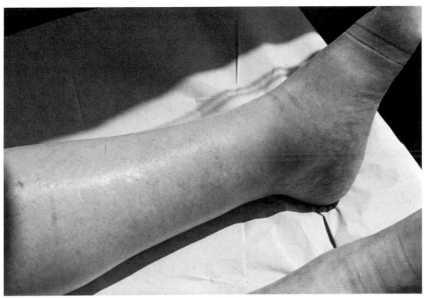

681

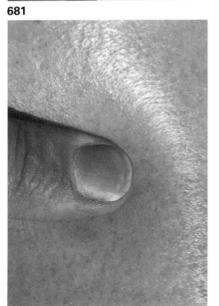

682

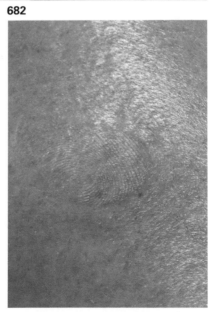

683 *Milroy's disease (lymphatic channel block)* Chronic long standing oedema with thickening of the sub-cutaneous tissues. In this congenital abnormality of the lymphatics the swelling is firmer, less easily displaced and therefore does not pit so well on pressure. Ulceration may occur. *(William Forsyth Milroy, 1855–1942, described 1891, New York.)*

684 *Filariasis of the leg (parasitic lymph block)* The oedema here is due to lymphatic blockage producing long standing firm oedema comparable to that of Milroy's disease. The filariae block the lymphatic channels.

685 *Rickets, active* There is swelling at the epiphyseal/metaphyseal junction at the knee due to a profusion of osteoid tissue.

683

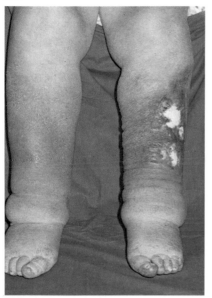

684

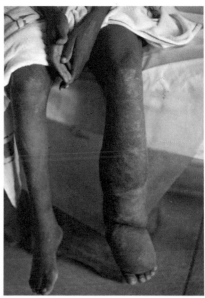

685

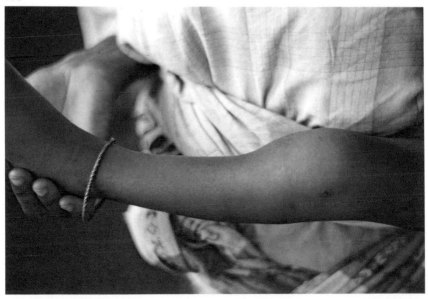

686 & 687 *Rickets, active* This swelling can be seen in the x-ray (**686**), and the changes of healing rickets with calcification seen in the following x-ray. Note that a bow-legged deformity has appeared.

688–690 *Rickets* The soft osteoid, which does not calcify, may be deformed by gravity and produce bowing, knock knee or other bizarre deformations of the limbs.

686

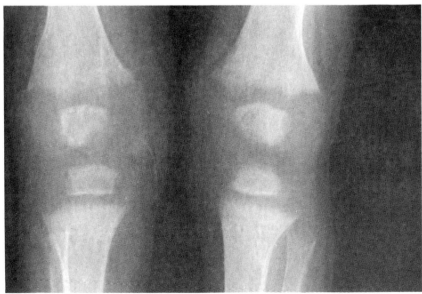

687

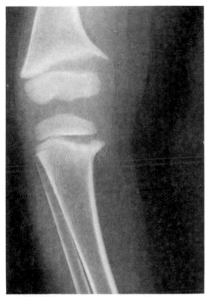

688

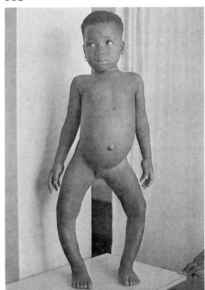

689

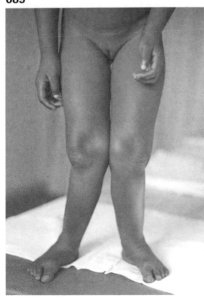

690

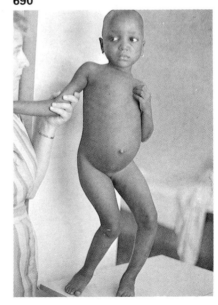

691 & 692 *Bowing of the tibia (tertiary yaws)* The anterior bowing or sabre like deformity of the tibia is secondary to a periostitis. (See x-ray). The leg itself remains straight and the thickening is on the anterior surface of the bone. A similar appearance may occur in the periostitis of syphilis. It should not be confused with the bowed tibia with curvature of the bone itself which is expanded and warm. This occurs in Paget's disease.

693 & 694 *Paget's disease (osteitis deformans)* Expansion and bowing of the tibia. *(Sir James Paget, 1814–1899, described 1877.)*

691

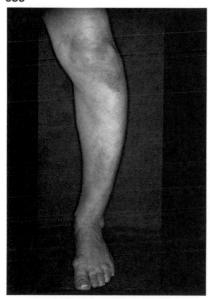

692

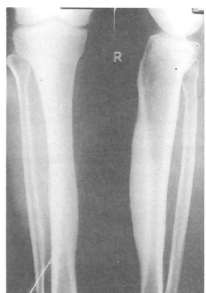

693

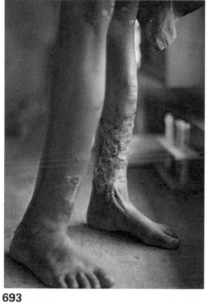

694

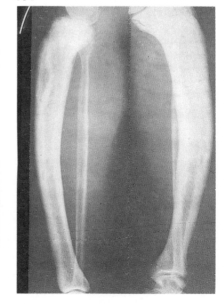

695 *Osteoarthritis, Baker's cyst* The bulge at the posterior lateral margin of the knee is caused by a herniation of synovium from the joint. It may only be noted when the knee is extended and may present with pain caused by rupture of the cyst. *(William Morrant Baker, 1839–1896, described 1885.)*

696–698 *Calloused knees* The weight is carried on the tibial tuberosities when kneeling on hard stone floors: a religious Russian lady (**696**).

The weight is carried onto the patella and above (**697**), when kneeling and then stretching forwards scrubbing the floor. This leads to supra patellar bursitis – house-maid's knee. Both the above may be seen in monumental brass enthusiasts – from kneeling and rubbing the brass.

The above must be differentiated from psoriasis (**698**) which has a predilection for the knee.

695

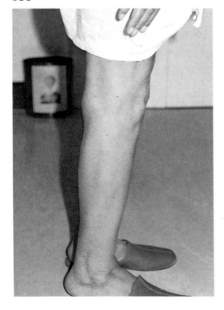

696

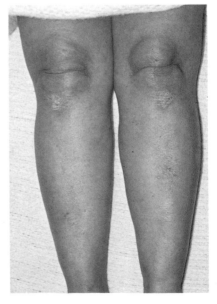

697

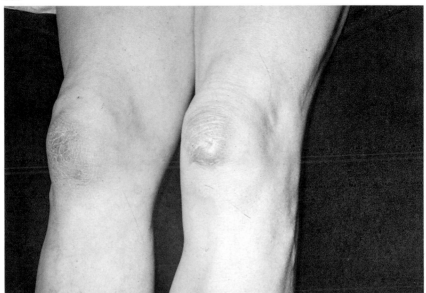

698

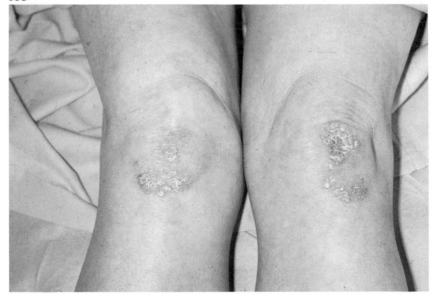

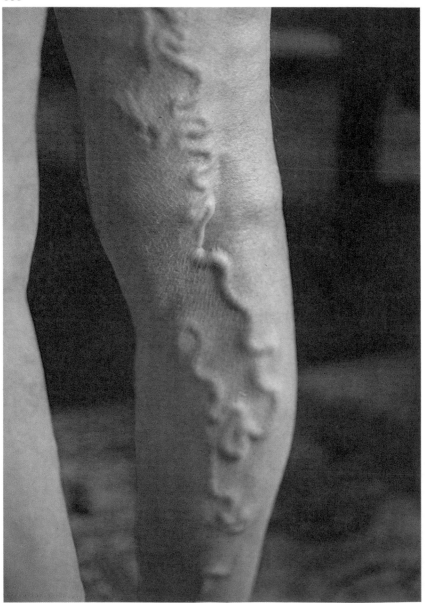

699 *Varicose veins* Tortuosity secondary to distension and secondary to valvular insufficiency. This leads to **700**, a surgical problem.

700 *Varicose eczema* The increased capillary pressure leads to a secondary itch and scratching and to the production of varicose eczema. The pigmentation is due to the deposition of haemosiderin in the tissues.

700

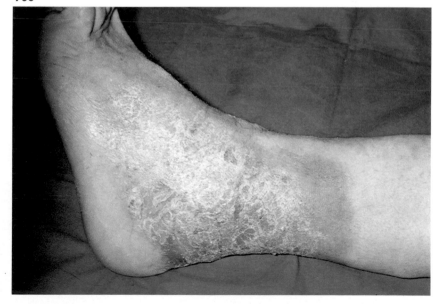

701 *Varicose ulcer* Eventually the skin may break down at the site of the eczema producing a characteristic ulcer usually in the lower third of the leg. Note the varicose veins, the eczema surrounding the ulcer and the slight oedema of the leg. The ulcer is clean with heavy granulation and a sharp margin which is not rolled. The pigmentation is due to the bandage which was applied prior to the photograph being taken.

Differential diagnosis of ulcers in the leg includes: (1) tropical ulcer – usually in the middle third; (2) congenital haemolytic anaemia; (3) syphilitic gummata; (4) haemoglobinopathies – sickle cell disease; (5) oedematous states with stasis; (6) arterial insufficiency; (7) neuropathy; (8) ulcerative colitis; (9) diabetes.

702 *Venous congestion* This woman had a large mass in her pelvis pressing on the veins and producing slight oedema of the right leg. This photograph shows slight puffiness of the right foot compared with the left. A venous block of minor degree in the pelvis may produce slight oedema of the leg and foot and the differential diagnosis between a deep venous thrombosis and a pelvic tumour may only be made after careful examination.

703 *Deep venous thrombosis* Slight puffiness of the leg with dilatation of the superficial veins as a secondary effect.

701

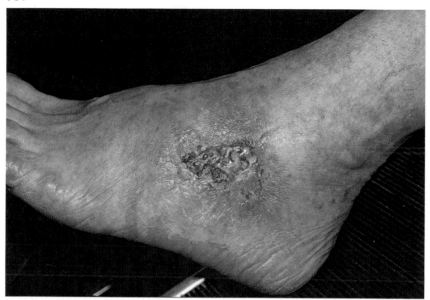

702

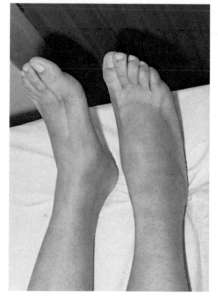

703

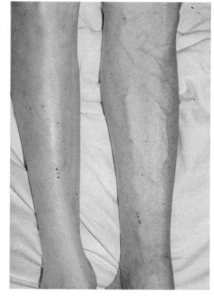

704

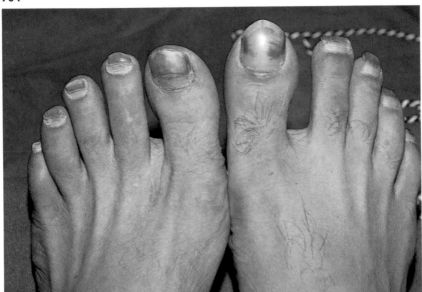

705

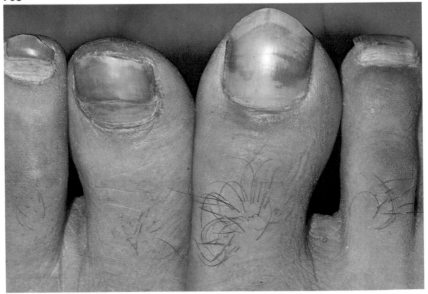

704 & 705 *Arterial insufficiency in the foot* Before the development of overt ischaemic signs the nutrition of the skin appendages is affected. The hair may become sparse and defects in nail growth may occur. The linear indentation running transversely was first described by Beau in 1846: it is due to interference with the nutrition of the nail and consequent depression of nail growth. The cause may be localised to the limb or related to systemic illness. See **531** for a full discussion.

706 *Gangrene of the toe* Once death takes place the tissue discolours, and the line of demarcation can be seen where there is a zone of erythema. This is the common picture in diabetic arteriopathy.

706

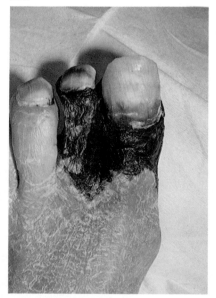

707 *Frost bite* Gangrene of all the toes secondary to exposure. This man spent the night sleeping on the London Embankment in the open and developed frost bite of the feet and gangrene of all the toes. The severity being aggravated by an impaired arterial circulation. The line of demarcation with the erythema can be seen particularly in the right toe. Subsequently he lost some of the toes but his functional feet were preserved.

707

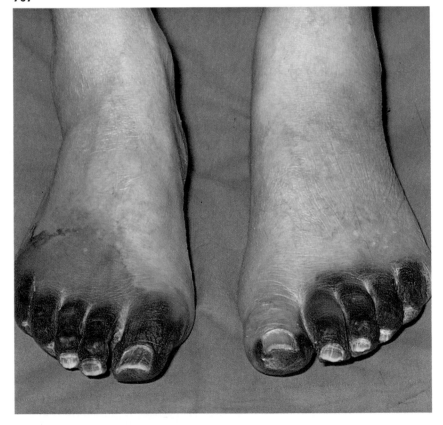

708 *Buerger's disease affecting hands and feet* This young male smoker with peripheral vascular insufficiency and thrombophlebitis with Raynaud's disease in the upper limb has lost the great toe of the left foot and there are trophic changes in the feet, trophic changes in the nail and a similar loss of digits in the hand due to arterial block. See **457.** *(Leo Buerger, 1879–1943, described 1908.)*

708

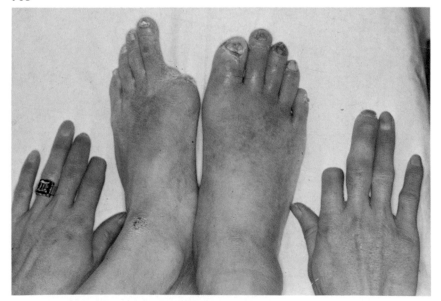

709 *Diabetic gangrene* A typical site in the diabetic, may be simple vascular insufficiency but usually a combination of poor blood supply, infection, neuropathy (poor sensation) – one of the three being dominant.

710 *Infected diabetic gangrene* If infection supervenes then the toe may be lost and infection spreads into the foot.

711 *Infected diabetic foot* No gross gangrene as such but a sinus is present and a chronic abscess is present in the web space.

712 *Diabetic gangrene, infection and neuropathy* All present in the same leg.

709

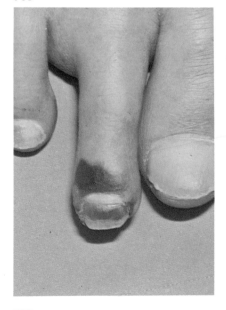

710

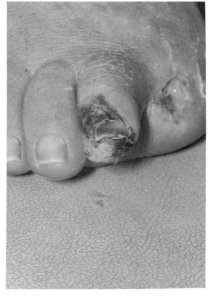

711

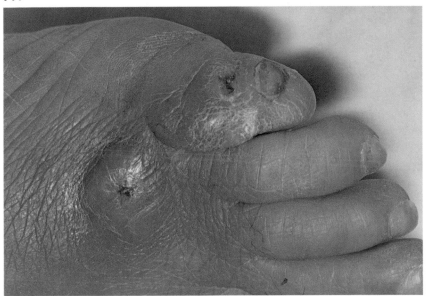

712

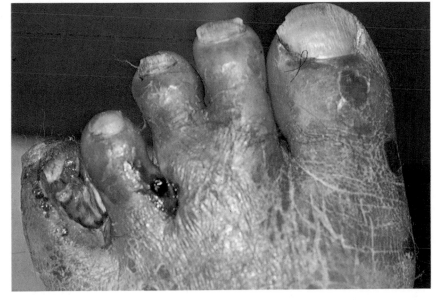

713 *Perforating ulcer of the foot* A trophic change occurring on the foot or heel related to loss of sensation. A perforating ulcer worms deep into the foot. Superficially not a lot may be seen (**714**). Perforating ulcers occur in neuropathic conditions such as diabetes, leprosy, and tabes dorsalis.

This patient had tuberculoid leprosy and in addition to the perforating ulcer had palpable nerves in the neck and on the back of the hand – plates **567** and **178**.

714 *Perforating ulcer (diabetic)* This man had peripheral neuropathy and was unable to appreciate pain. A slight swelling of the foot due to infection developed but he continued to walk on it. When the hard skin at the base of the toe was removed a deep penetrating ulcer extending into the phalanx was present. Note the dried up gangrenous tip to the second toe.

715 *Cellulitis of the foot (diabetic)* The blood supply is good but there is a neuropathy and infection. Beau's lines are present on the great toenail and superficial gangrene has developed between the fourth and fifth toes due to the pressure produced by poorly fitting pointed shoes pressing the toes together.

716 *Arterial embolus* Embolus in the popliteal fossa. Initially the leg becomes painful, pale, paralysed, then pulseless. It progresses to gangrene as is seen here.

713

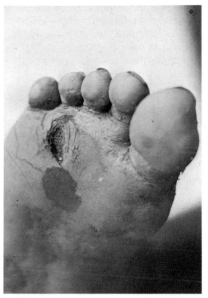

714

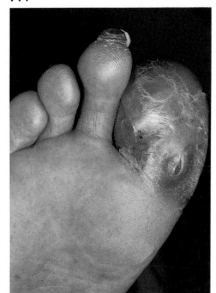

715

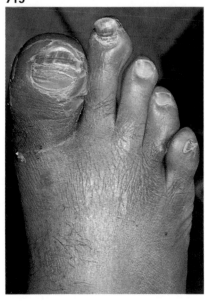

716

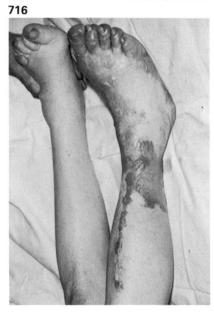

717 *Saddle embolus at the aortic bifurcation (gas gangrene)* No pulses below the aorta. Gas is present in the muscle and delineates the septa producing a feathery appearance. A young Nigerian male was brought by his friends to casualty. He was unable to walk and was very ill and anxious.

Two days earlier he had suddenly developed pain and paralysis in the legs. A native medicine man was summoned who excoriated the limbs and rubbed in a powder of dung, earth and leaves. He did not improve and came, as a last resort, to hospital. He died.

718 *Bacterial endocarditis* Small emboli trapped in the skin. Emboli of this size are difficult to distinguish from purpura.

719 *Pressure sore on the heel* This sore in a diabetic is due to the pressure produced by a tight shoe: friction produces an ulcer.

720 *A bed sore* Note the site of the sore is over the point of the heel since the pressure is related to the bed. Compare this with the previous plate where the pressure is over the insertion of the achilles tendon and the pressure is due to the rim of the shoe.

The early signs of a pressure sore – initial redness proceeding to stasis and discoloration due to the impairment of circulation. It may develop within the space of a night if the foot is not regularly moved. The bed sores occur over the great trochanter, between the knees, over the sacrum and buttocks and on the back of the ribs (**618**).

717

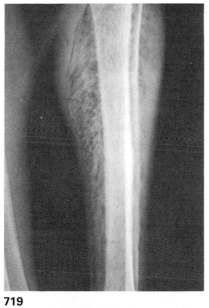

718

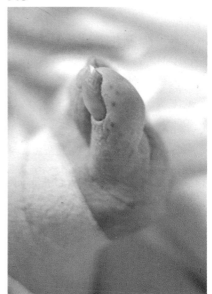

719

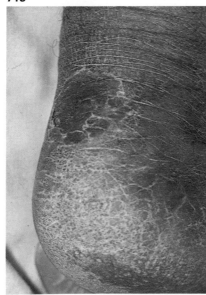

720

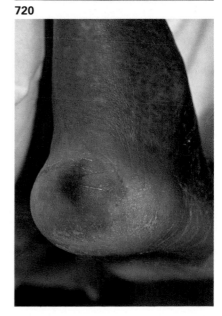

721 *Quadriceps wasting (polio)* Muscle wasting is a common physical sign of disuse. It occurs: rapidly with bed rest even of short duration and will be symmetrical; after injury, on that side; after denervation, lower motor neurone, as in polio. Upper motor neurone lesions by comparison produce little wasting.

A lower motor neurone lesion in childhood leads to growth impairment and a disparity in length of the limbs.

722 *Poliomyelitis affecting the right leg* Note the difference in size, the asymmetrical muscle wasting and the shortness of the femur.

723 & 724 *Tabes dorsalis, neuropathic joint* There is asymmetrical quadriceps wasting secondary to disuse, and a Charcot's joint at the left knee. The leg is supported by a caliper. The knee was painless and demonstrates (**724**) an abnormal range of movement. Neuropathic joints may occur in any situation where the pain sensation is diminished. Diabetes, leprosy, and tabes are common causes. Infection and sinus formation may occur. *(Jean Martine Charcot, 1825–1893, French neurologist, described 1868.)*

721

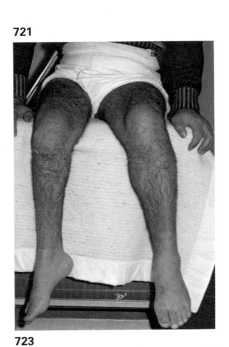

722

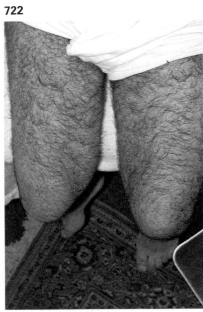

723

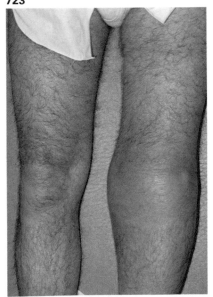

724

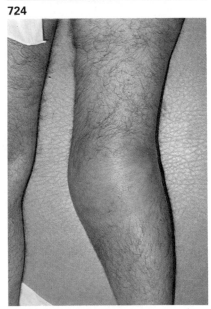

725 *Tabes dorsalis* Diminished pain sensation. The patient was having physiotherapy to improve muscle power and heat as a placebo for her lightning pains. She persuaded the physiotherapist to give her more and more heat, she was aware of the warm sensation but felt no pain and sustained a burn. The patient with a neuropathy is in grave danger from hot water bottles and appliances that emit heat.

726 *Clawing of the toes* Due to a disturbance in muscle balance in the foot. It may be associated with pes cavus, and be familial and present from birth. There is an association with Friedreich's ataxia and peroneal muscular atrophy. *(Nikolas Friedreich, 1825–1882, described 1863.)*

727 *Clawed toes* Your thought association pattern should include: is there a family history of ataxia or is there kyphoscoliosis? ═ Friedreich's ataxia. Is there bilateral foot drop or wasting to the knees? ═ peroneal muscular atrophy.

728 *Hallux valgus* The deviation of the great toe laterally with the pro-minence of the metacarpo-phalangeal joint on the medial side of the foot may be associated with pain and with swelling and discomfort, particularly if a bunion forms over it as has happened in this case: differentiate it from an acute monoarthritis.

725

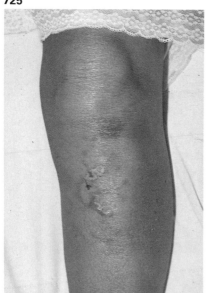

726

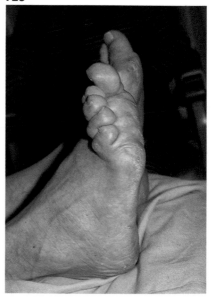

727

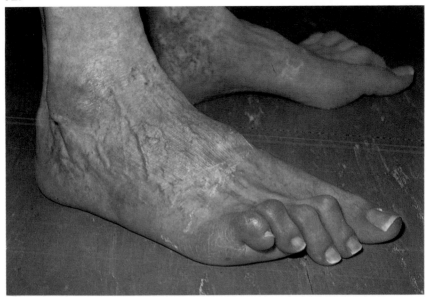

728

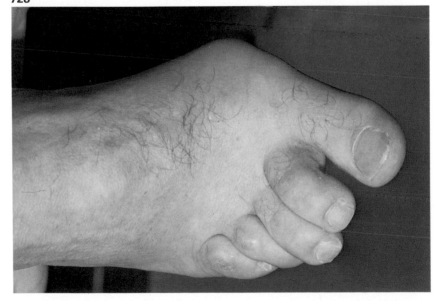

729 *The extensor plantar response (Babinski response)* The classic sign of an upper motor neurone lesion. Suspect it when testing tone by rolling the leg (external/internal rotation at the hip). Elicit it with a blunt, pointed object – a key – by stroking firmly the lateral edge of the foot (warn the patient): watch closely. In an early lesion the up-going toe may only appear once or twice and then you will be in the doubtful area of 'The plantars are equivocal!' The gross extensor plantar is demonstrated in this picture. It may also be elicited by firm pressure on the shin and a down stroke to the foot (Oppenheim's sign). The extensor plantar means a pyramidal tract lesion. Next look for a level; remember that a lesion could be anywhere from the motor cortex to the anterior horn cell. Don't x-ray the lumbar spine as your first investigation, the cord stops at the first lumbar vertebra. Look for reflex changes – if the leg tendon reflexes are absent the cord lesion must be combined with a neuropathy. Absent ankle jerks with up-going toes occur in (1) taboparesis, (2) Friedreich's ataxia, (3) subacute combined degeneration of the cord, (4) a conus or lower cord lesion. Conversely, absent ankle jerks and down-going toes mean a neuropathy or an L5 S1 root lesion. *(Joseph Francois Felix Babinski, 1857–1932; Hermann Oppenheim, 1858–1919.)*

730 *Hyperkeratosis of the feet (practolol)* This may be due to: (1) friction and walking bare foot; (2) as part of tylosis – a congenital defect associated with hyperkeratosis of the palms and carcinoma of the oesophagus; (3) as a drug reaction: e.g. practolol; (4) with psoriasis.

731 *Melanoma in an Arab* A melanoma may be seen in any site in the European – it may be a pigmented or non-pigmented primary. In Arabia a primary melanoma other than a subungual or plantar one is exceedingly uncommon.

729

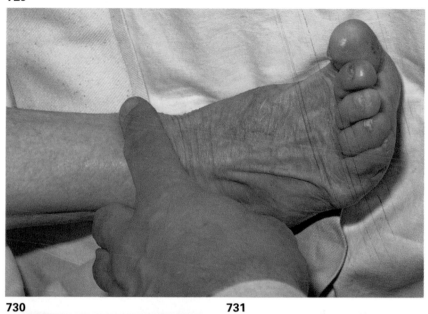

730

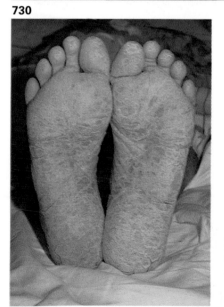

731

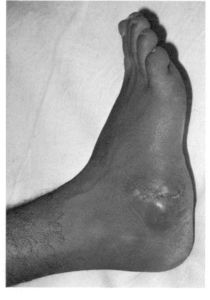

732

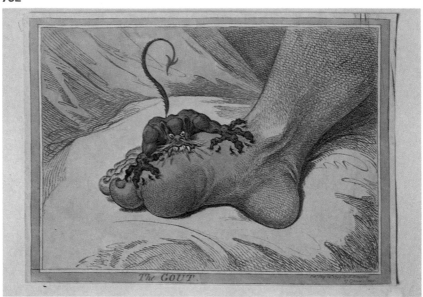

The GOUT.

733

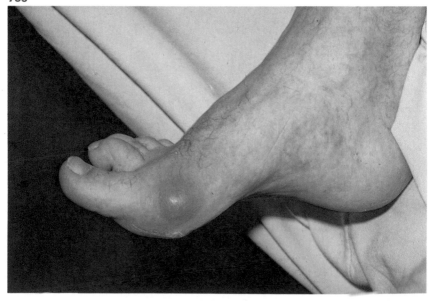

732 *Gout and the feet (Podagra: Gk podos, foot; agra, trap)* The classic view of gout enshrined in James Gilray's late 18th century cartoon and in subsequent Punch cartoons of the late 19th and early 20th centuries of rich fat old men who drank port in their clubs with a bandaged foot put up on a gout stool. But gout affects any joint, usually as a monoarthritis – thumb, wrist or knee as well as the predilection for the great toe which may be related to the trauma and early osteoarthritis that may affect it.

733 *Acute gout* A hot, red, very tender MP joint of the great toe coming on *acutely* in a man who had had a laparotomy. Acute gout has a tendency to flare up post-operatively. An inflamed bunion can look identical. Subsequently the foot became more swollen and then after two days gradually subsided.

734 *Gout* At the end of a long drawn out attack the skin may peel.

735 *Chronic tophaceous gout* It bears a superficial resemblance to acute infection.

734

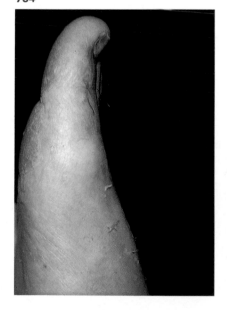

735

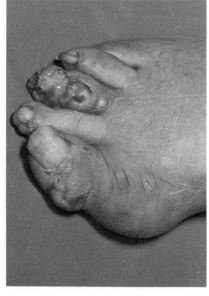

736 *'Nigra onychia'* Ruba onychia (nail varnish) descends from the need for the women to demonstrate to the male which of them were available and which were menstruating. Nigra onychia is the result of soaking the feet in a patent medicine containing potassium permanganate.

This man (a publican who drank excessive alcohol) developed burning feet and alcoholic hepatitis (**796**). His doctor arranged an out-patient appointment three weeks hence at a liver unit, meanwhile the feet became unbearable. He therefore sat drinking in the evening with his feet in the patent medicine – the potassium permanganate reacted with the keratin and dyed the skin dark brown. Before his appointment he scrubbed off the skin but could not dislodge the potassium permanganate from the nails. Hence nigra onychia.

A silly story – but the patient went to the MRCP examination and though the abdomen showed hepatosplenomegaly and a liver biopsy puncture, the nails caused a lot of anxious moments to the candidates. Always get the patient's confidence and he will tell you the answers.

737 *Ainhum* Aetiology unknown. Common in West Africa amongst those who go barefoot. An initial constriction at the base of the little toe tightens like a tourniquet and ultimately the toe falls off or is knocked off. Treatment is to amputate – the next toe may be involved. The pathology is just fibrous tissue at the base of the toe. There is no neurological or vascular defect nor systemic illness.

738 *Guinea worm (dracunculus medinensis)* The female worm has succeeded in its life aim and come to the point of egg laying. A blister forms at the foot, ruptures and in response to contact with water discharges a white fluid – the larvae – these then make for the secondary host, the crustacean Cyclops, and the cycle begins again. The worms may get lost and are often noted curled up and calcified on x-rays or felt beneath the skin (**634**). They have a predilection to come out on skin which is in contact with water. Treatment consists of winding them out a little at a time onto a stick and facilitating this by bathing with water. If the worm is broken (they may be up to 30 inches long) acute inflammation develops. Niridazole orally will allow the worm to be withdrawn easily.

736

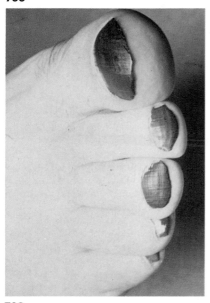

737

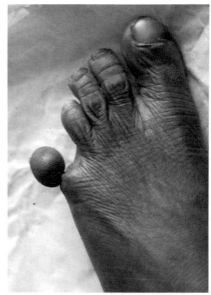

738

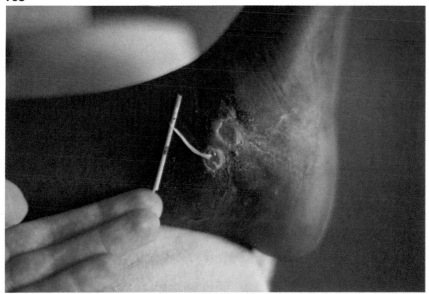

Dermatology and General Medicine

No attempt has been made to cover dermatology but a few common skin conditions are illustrated.

739 *Chickenpox* A rash is present over the chest of a child. Macules, papules, vesicles and crusts are seen, the rash is therefore in varying stages of development, i.e. polymorphic. It is evenly spread over the chest and less on the limbs, i.e. centripetal. The white substance is Calamine lotion.

740 *Chickenpox* The distribution of the rash of chickenpox tends to be centripetal over the trunk. This appearance may be modified since the rash appears to come out most profusely over those areas which are either warmer, moister or not exposed to light. In this baby the rash has been most prominent in the napkin area. It is not a nappy rash *per se* since it affects the skin creases which would normally be protected from the nappy and its chemical decomposition products. The rash is generalised, there are sparse spots seen on the trunk. All stages are present from macule to vesicle.

741 *Chickenpox enanthem* The chickenpox vesicles will also be present inside the mouth and appear as small aphthae.

739

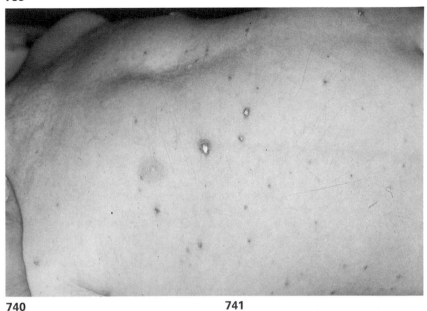

740

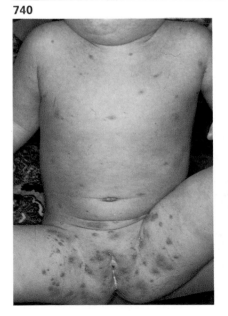

741

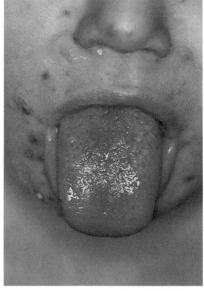

742 *Chickenpox* The all important differential diagnosis of chickenpox is smallpox. Smallpox cannot be diagnosed as chickenpox. The essential difference is (1) *distribution,* (2) *the speed of evolution of the rash.* Umbilication and rash on the palms of the hands are unreliable differential points. The most important factor is the overall distribution pattern, even though there may be few spots.

On the shoulder of this African child can be seen vesicles, macules, papules and one crust. A polymorphic rash is highly suggestive of chickenpox but to make the diagnosis one would have to consider the overall distribution of the rash. Bear in mind that smallpox tends to affect those areas exposed to light and air and will even be more prominent over bony prominences such as the skin, malleoli, supraorbital ridges and nose.

743 *Smallpox* The classic rash: vesicular, profuse, almost confluent with umbilication. All the vesicles are at the same stage of evolution. Note the increase in rash over the face and arms; the sparseness over the trunk can be seen in the right hand corner of the photograph. This distribution is much the most important criterion for diagnosis.

742

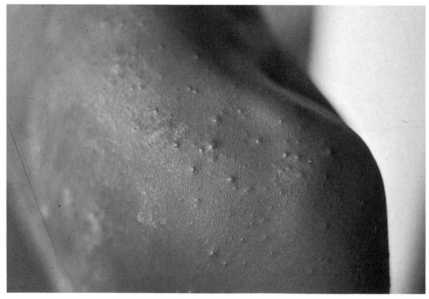

743

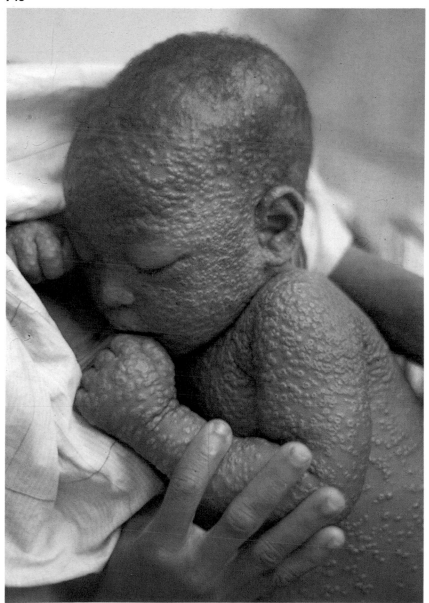

744 *The distribution of mild smallpox* The distribution of the sparse spots are seen over the trunk, more profuse over the limbs where the rash tends to be at the same stage of evolution. There is also some rash over the face but the child has moved just as the picture was taken.

745 *Mild smallpox* The rash is present over the face, trunk and arms in all stages of evolution though there is tendency for the rash to be in the early vesicular stage. It is more marked over the face and tends to be particularly pronounced over the nose, malar regions and the cheeks, sparing the inner margins of the eye and the axillae.

746 *Mild smallpox* Note the rash across the eyebrow and down the bridge of the nose sparing the inside corner of the eye covering the chin and tending to spare the upper lip.

747 *Smallpox, healed* This healed smallpox rash demonstrates one characteristic of smallpox, it spares the axilla.

748 *Mild smallpox* A pleomorphic rash.

744

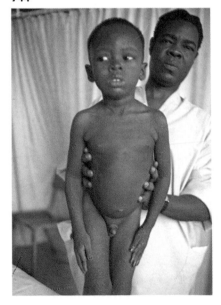

745

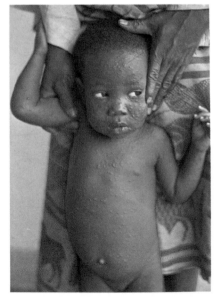

746

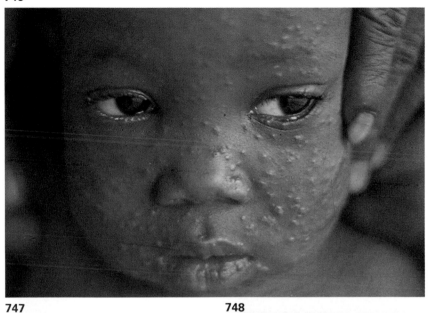

747

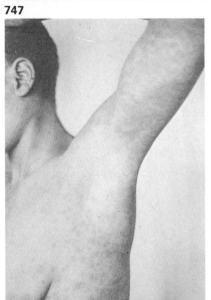

748

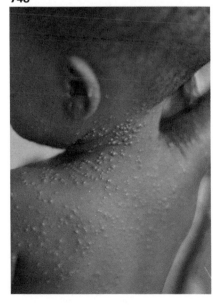

749 *A smallpox vaccination* A good clean primary vaccination just beginning to scab.

Smallpox revaccination protects against three characteristics of the disease, toxaemia, the number of the spots and their character. The development will be modified, the one thing that does tend to remain the same is the distribution. Remember the vaccination scar can occur in modified smallpox. It is essential to consider the distribution and the speed of development; always diagnose smallpox rather than chickenpox if there is any doubt.

750 *Smallpox vaccination* The red line of lymphangitis up the arm to the elbow. An extensive erythematous oedematous area is present around the vaccination. Previous vaccination had been performed five years earlier.

751 & 752 *Smallpox vaccination in a patient on prednisone* Evolution in the vaccination. Note the spread over the chest and breast. It is most important to consider the contra-indications to vaccination before revaccination is performed. The absolute contra-indications are: (1) eczema, (2) blood dyscrasia, (3) immunosuppression, or (4) steroid therapy.

749

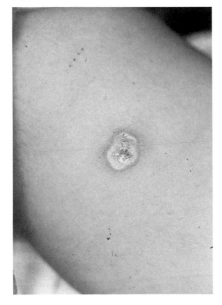

750

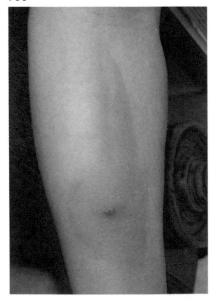

751

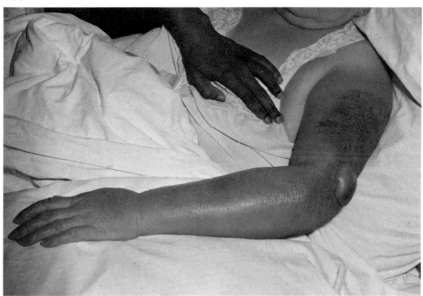

752

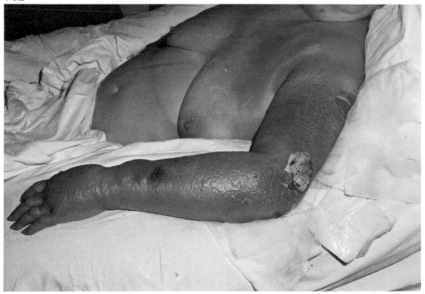

753 *Measles (morbilli)* The child is miserable and unhappy, reverting to suckling at its mother's breast. There is a mild conjunctivitis and an early macular papular rash is just visible on the forehead.

754 *Koplik's spots* In the mouth the spots may be seen as white grains on a red background.

753

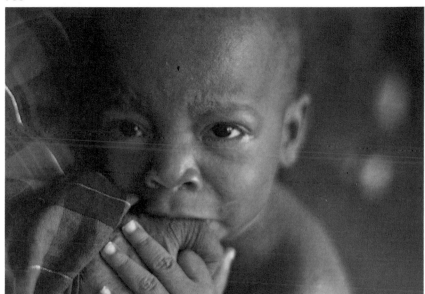

754

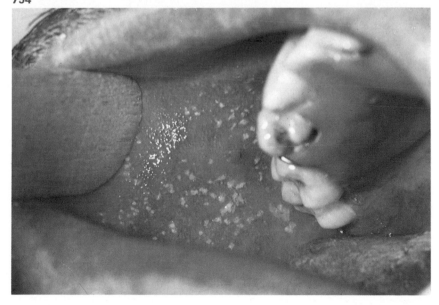

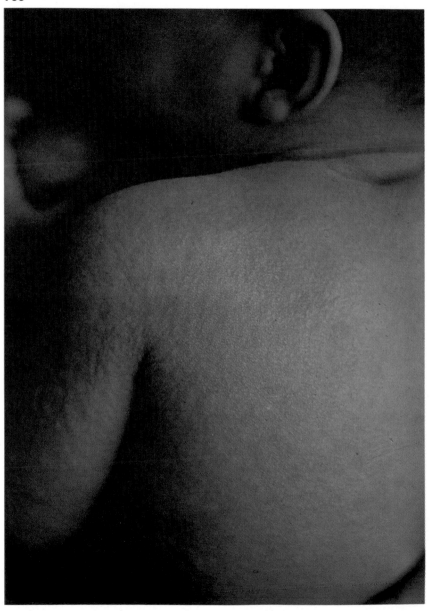

755 *Measles (morbilli)* A profuse macular papular rash can be seen over the back. Papules coalesce producing a thick furry appearance to the skin and a dark red colour which comes through the normal skin pigmentation. In the lower part of the back the normal skin can be seen between the rash.

756 *Measles rash, European* The colour of the rash can be appreciated in the child with measles.

756

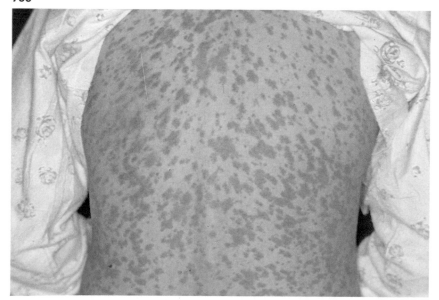

757 *Desquamating measles rash* An extreme example.

758 *Measles* After five or six days the rash starts to flake and a browny desquamation occurs. If this is severe huge plaques of skin can flake off. Note the angular stomatitis present.

759 *Rubella* The rashes produced by viral infections tend to be similar in appearance. It is easy to mistake German measles for another virus infection such as infectious mononucleosis. If it is also complicated by an arthritis it may be confused with mumps or viral hepatitis. The rash is maculo-papular with sparse spots from 1–4mm in diameter. It appears first on the cheeks, spreads onto the trunk and limbs remaining discrete. Lymph node enlargement is a constant finding but the mucous membranes of the mouth are clean compared with the redness seen in measles. A few flecks of exudate may be seen on the tonsils. Conjunctivae may be a faint pink rather than the acute conjunctivitis of measles.

757

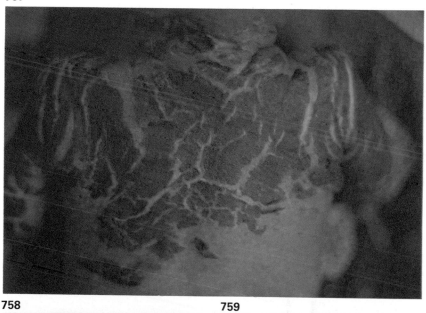

758

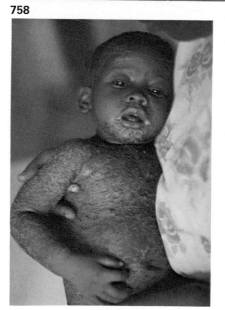

759

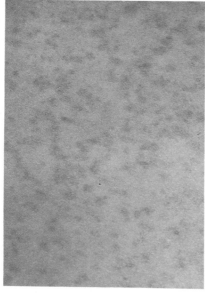

760

761

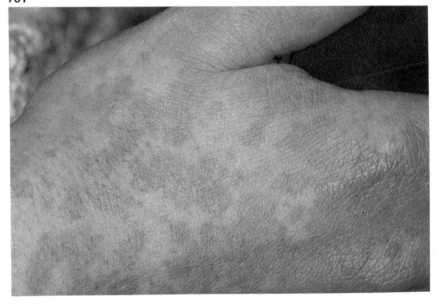

760 *Rubella* Larger macules and papules on the limbs.

761 *Infectious mononucleosis* The rash induced by Ampicillin in infectious mononucleosis for comparison with that due to German measles. It is easy to confuse infectious mononucleosis and German measles (rubella).

762 & 763 *Rubella polyarthritis* 15% of adults with rubella may develop arthritis which appears about one week after the rash (affecting the fingers, wrists, elbows and knees without systemic upset). The attacks may persist up to twenty eight days. They are self limiting and leave no residue – **763**, hand and wrist one week later.

Viral diseases such as dengue, mumps, smallpox and viral hepatitis as well as virus vaccines may produce a similar arthropathy.

762

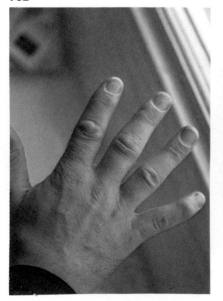

763

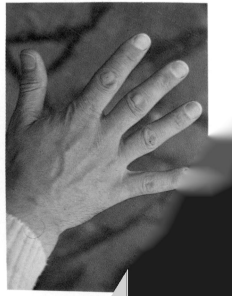

764 *Senile hyperkeratosis* Brown raised hyperpigmented patches occurring with age and associated with exposure to sunlight. It is important to be aware of the development of basal cell carcinoma amongst the hyperkeratotic areas. The senile keratosis itself is a non-malignant condition and the commonest benign tumour of the skin in the elderly.

765 *Erythema ab igne* Seen in winter, usually in women. From it can be deduced the side of the fire on which the patient sits! There is an erythema combined with browny discoloration related to change in the haemoglobin in the skin. Removal from the source of heat gradually produces clearing of the lesion.

Pityriasis

There are four common conditions characterised by a branny desquamation (pityriasis, Gk *bran*) : P. rosea, P. capitus (dandruff), P. rubra (exfoliative dermatitis), and P. versicolor (tinea versicolor).

766 & 767 *Pityriasis versicolor (a yeast infection)* This infection of the skin is extremely common and shows up particularly during the summer when the affected skin is paler than the normal skin. Its patches may persist for years and on closer examination they are observed to be perifollicular in distribution. These patches may coalesce and have a velvety surface with scales which can be scraped off. They must not be confused with vitiligo. Pityriasis versicolor itches, vitiligo does not.

764

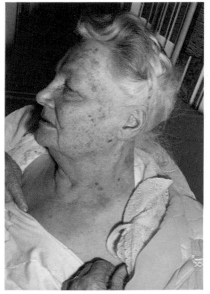

765

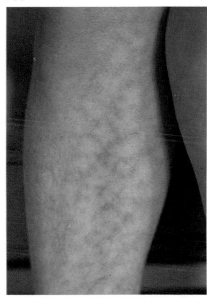

766

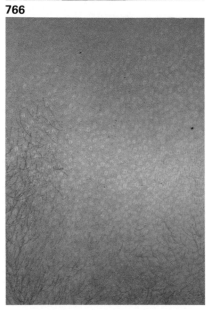

767

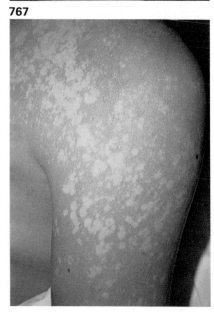

768–771 *Pityriasis rosea* The maculo-papular rash is usually limited to the trunk. An initial large 'herald' patch may precede the main rash by a week to ten days (**768**). The lesions, round and nummular have an erythematous edge and central branny desquamation (**769, 771**). They tend to follow the cleavage lines of the skin (**770**). The condition lasts about six weeks and clears spontaneously.

768

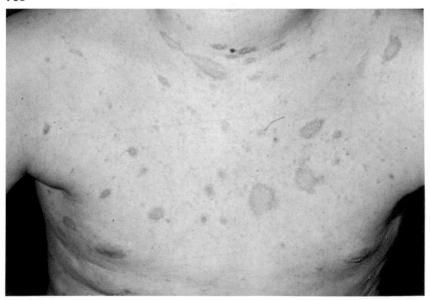

769

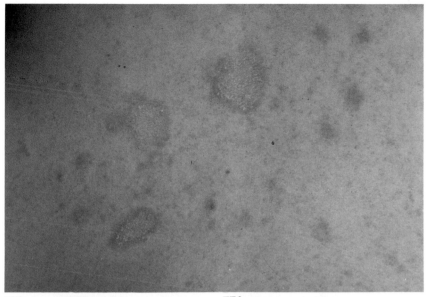

770

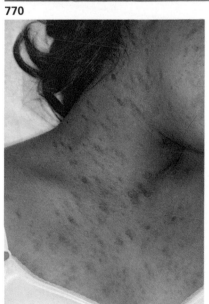

771

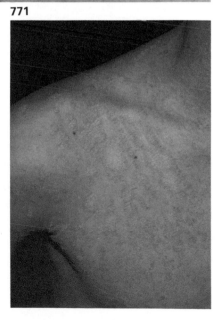

Erythema multiforme

A common skin disease. Begins as an erythematous plaque 0.5–1cm in diameter which progresses to bulla formation (cause is unknown) often associated with streptococcal infection, occasionally with underlying neoplasm and may recur after attacks of herpes simplex. Sometimes a drug is incriminated. Minor attacks clear spontaneously but severe attacks may be accompanied with toxicity and require steroids. A variant with involvement of mucous membranes occurs particularly in children – Stevens-Johnson syndrome. *(Albert Mason Stevens, New York paediatrician, 1884–1945, described 1922; Frank Chambliss Johnson, 1894–1934.)*

772 *Erythema multiforme* Characteristic target lesions or erythema iris. Two weeks previously the man had had a herpes simplex infection of the penis. (See **239**).

773 *Erythema multiforme, target lesions* The target lesions or erythema iris – a central vesicle with a clear area and an erythematous ring around it. The lesions may vary from vesicles bullae to macules and papules. Erythema multiforme tends to look like this but 'multiforme' is a little misleading.

772

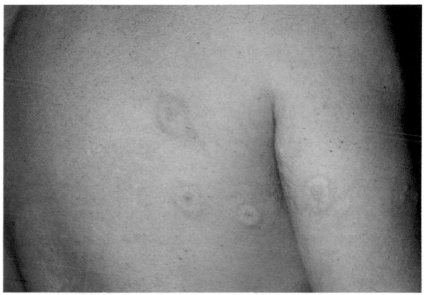

773

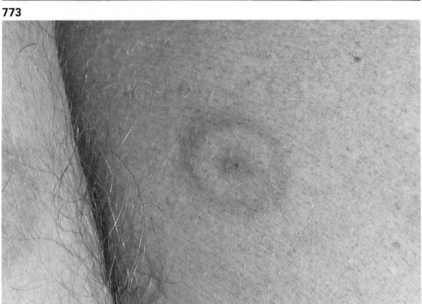

774 *Erythema multiforme* An ageing lesion in erythema multiforme with some haemorrhage into the vesicles.

775 *Stevens-Johnson syndrome* Erythema multiforme affecting the skin and mucous membranes can be life threatening. It can affect all the mucous membranes.

Skin manifestations which may be suggestive of an underlying malignant disease: (1) severe intractable itching (prurigo); (2) urticaria; (3) dermatitis herpetiformis, **(776)**; (4) acanthosis nigricans, **(777)**; (5) erythema multiforme, **(774)**; (6) hyperkeratosis palmaris, **(532)**.

776 *Dermatitis herpetiformis* Clusters of small itchy blisters, superficially akin to herpes simplex, occur on the face, shoulders, sacral area, elbows and knees. Associated with small bowel malabsorption and in the elderly there may be an underlying malignancy.

774

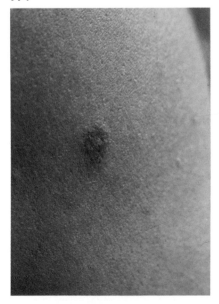

775

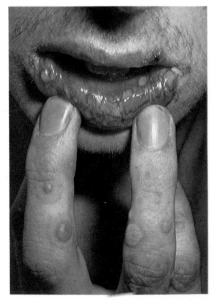

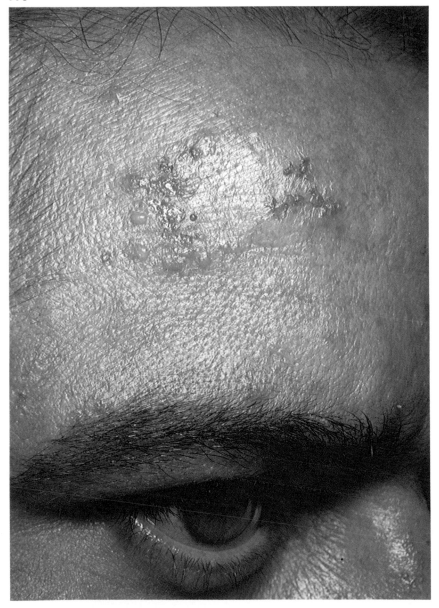

777 *Acanthosis nigricans* (1) *Juvenile type:* no association with malignancy. (2) *Adult type:* associated with malignancy. The skin is grey brown/dark brown in colour and becomes thickened, rugose and velvety. It may itch: warty excrescences vary from pin head to small pea size. It affects the back of the neck, perianal and genito crural flexures.

778 *Dermatomyositis* Classic heliotrope colour affecting the eyelids. Alleged association with malignant disease.

779 *Erythema nodosum* The nodules, found on the anterior surface of the shins and thighs, are raised, red, tender lumps 2–4cm in diameter which gradually flatten and then go through the spectrum of colour changes of a bruise from red, blue, yellow, green or black to normal. Associated with this may be an arthralgia and fever. Erythema nodosum is associated with acute streptococcal infection, rheumatic fever, primary tuberculosis, acute sarcoidosis, sulphonamides and pregnancy.

780 *Erythema nodosum* Evolving changes: note the lesions in the lower third of the right leg and in the middle third of the left shin.

777

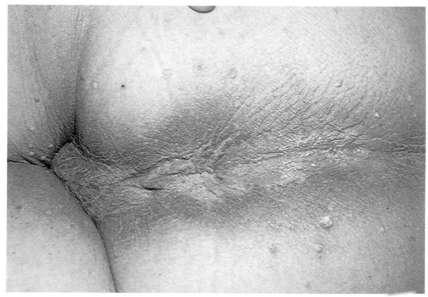

778

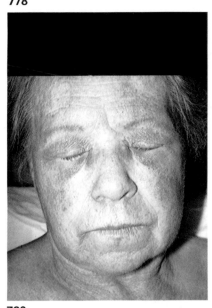

779

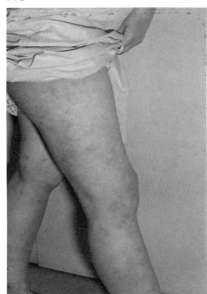

780

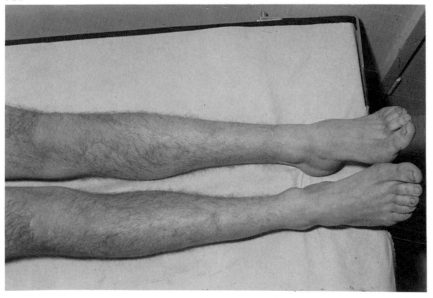

781–784 *Purpura* Characterised by blood in the skin producing purple spots varying from a pin head in size (petechiae as are seen here) through to large bruises (**782**). The purpura may be due to a deficiency of platelets – thrombocytopaenic purpura (**783**) or to capillary defect, as in Henoch-Schönlein purpura. Morphologically there is no difference, they both consist of blood in the skin.

Purpura does not blanch on pressure. Purpura also occurs in scurvy (capillary fragility), in old people (inelastic skin) as well as in patients on steroids and anticoagulants. It is more common on the legs. (Increased hydrostatic pressure – a physiological tourniquet test, **784**.) Figure **784** shows a gross ecchymosis in a patient on anticoagulants. *(Heinrich Eduard Henoch, 1820–1910, described 1868; Johann Lukas Schönlein, 1793–1864, described 1832.)*

781

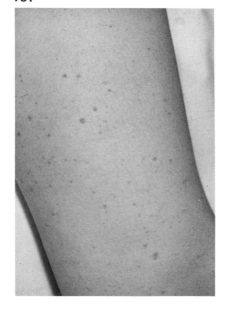

782

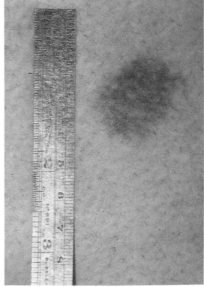

783

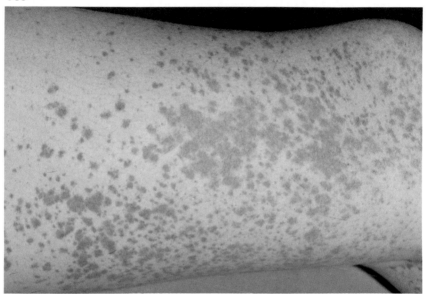

784

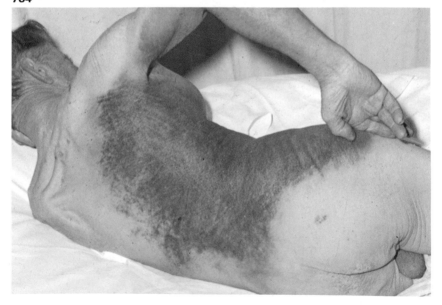

Appendix: The Significance of Callosities, Burns and Tattoos

This section is included in order to stimulate an interest in changes which may give a clue to disease or an insight into the patient's occupation or habits.

785 & 786 *Occupational callosities of the hand* Occupational callosities as opposed to the plain horny, hardened hands of the manual labourer may give insight or allow one to pick up extra information. Many have been described, two are illustrated.

There is a plaque of hardened skin on the lateral aspect of the terminal IP joint of the ring finger (*arrow*). This man was a businessman from Sarawak who did not indulge in manual labour. His passion was golf and the plaque was due to clutching the golf club as shown in **786**.

787 *Guitar callus* Callosities of the finger tip in a professional guitar player. They are due to the pressure of the fingers on the strings.

788 *Prayer callus* The Moslem priest prays assiduously several times a day, prayer involving the forehead touching the ground. This man – one of a group visiting this country, in common with his colleagues, had a callosity on his forehead from many years of prayer (*arrowed*).

785

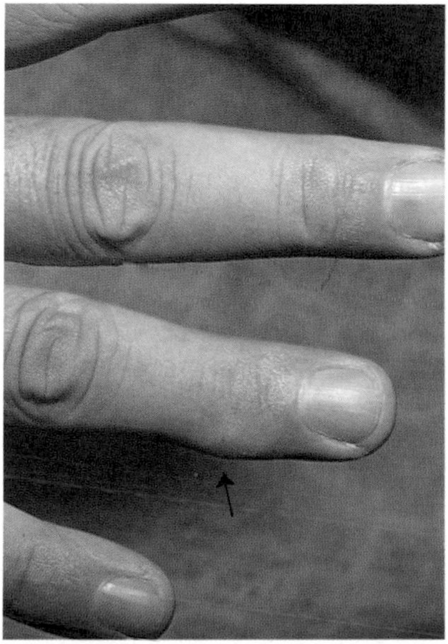

786

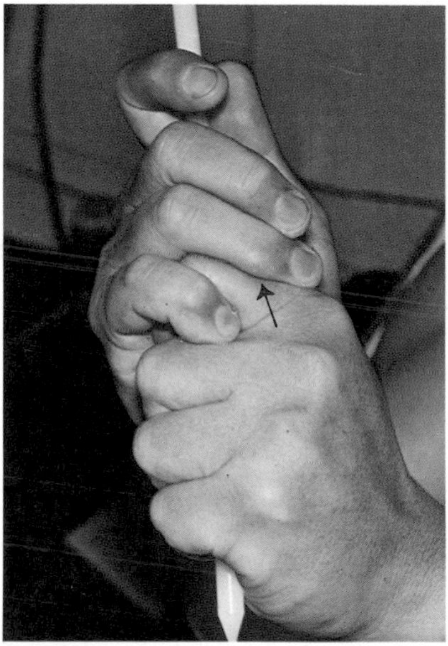

787

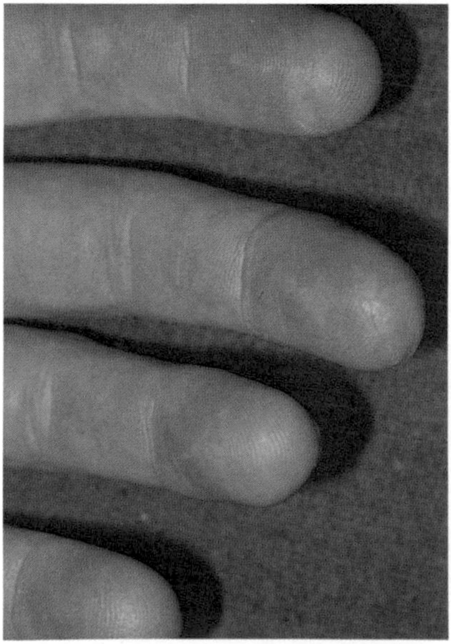

788

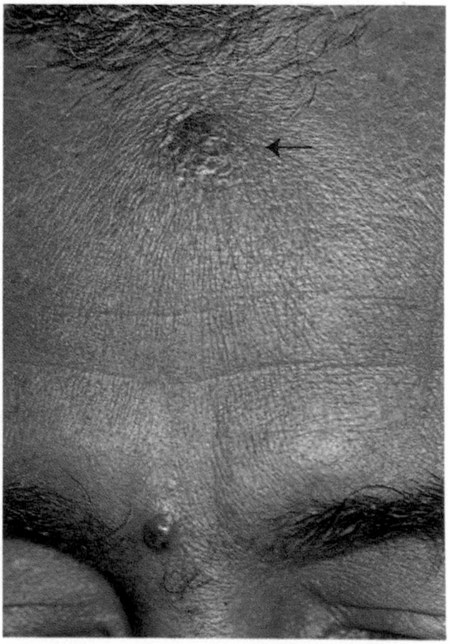

789 *Callus on the malleolus* In the Middle East the callosity on the outer border of the foot and the malleolus is a common feature and is due to the habit of sitting crosslegged with the foot tucked in under the buttock where it bears the weight against the ground.

790 *Occupational callosities* Repeated dorsiflexion of the foot in a chauffeur and the callus produced by rubbing against the tongue of his shoe.

791 *Tattoos and drug addiction* Repeated venepuncture leads to tattooing of the skin over the veins of the hands and wrists in a heroin addict. Tattooing of the skin for decorative purposes may be associated with an increased instance of hepatitis, dermal sensitivity to pigment and specific disease.

792 *Coal mining* This man presented with cough and breathlessness. The intradermal implantation of coal in a man who long ago gave up coal mining gives the clue to his previous occupation (*arrow*).

793 *Alcoholism* Classical cigarette burn occurring after falling into a deep alcoholic sleep.

789

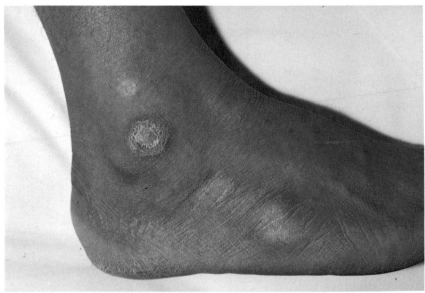

790

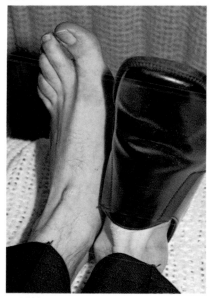

791

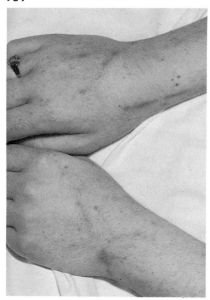

792

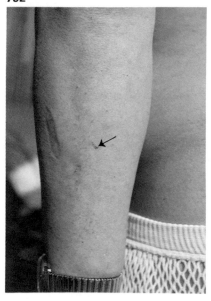

793

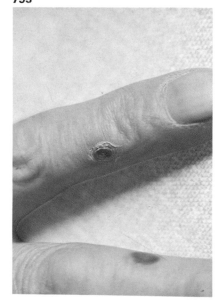

445

794 & 795 *Alcoholism* Another example of a cigarette burn in an alcoholic. A common occurrence in alcoholism which should alert one to the diagnosis. Turning the hand over reveals patchy palm erythema in this man who was complaining of burning feet and had erythromelalgia and 'liver soles' (**796**).

796 *Alcoholic cirrhosis* Note the erythema, analogous to palmar erythema, occurring in the feet.

797 *Henna staining on the hand* See below.

798 & 799 *Cigarette smoking* 60 cigarettes a day produces obvious staining, even 5–10 cigarettes a day can be smelt on the fingers. Staining of the palm may occur in cigarette smokers particularly if the cigarette is held with the ignited end between the fingers pointing into the palm where the smoke can drift out of the hollow and stain it. A similar palm staining is seen after the use of Henna as a cosmetic (**797**), this may be a deliberate result of staining the hands for the cosmetic effect or follow on dyeing the hair with henna before allowing it to dry in the sun. Smoothing it on and washing it off the hands still leaves yellow staining (see carotene colouring, **54**).

794

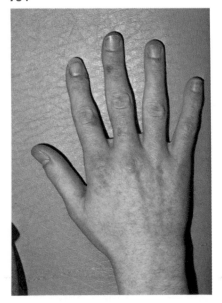

795

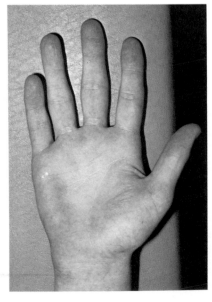

796

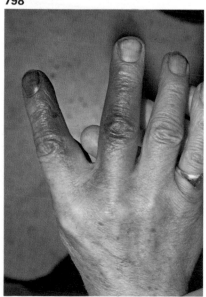

797

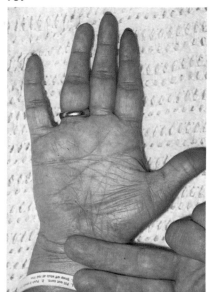

798

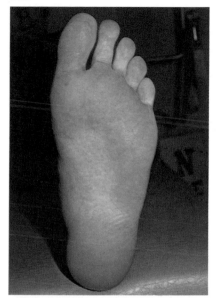

799

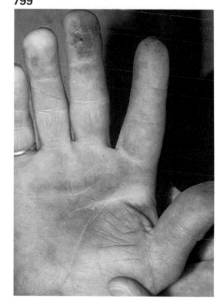

800 *The cautery (used as a powerful counter irritant)* The hand is one of the sites for the touch of the cautery in primitive medicine. The cautery burn or scar will be seen firstly over the sites of the maximum pain where it is used as a counter irritant and as such is a guide to the presence of pain or previous attacks of pain. It is also commonly placed on the head and on the limbs in small children for the treatment of the fevers of childhood. These methods of treatment are now seen world wide as immigrants and visitors who may have had these treatments years ago consult their doctors. The scars may lead to confusion on the part of the physician.

The cautery of the hand must be recognised as a burn and not confused with a squamous cell carcinoma (**801**).

801 *Squamous cell carcinoma* The squamous cell carcinoma of the skin in an Australian engineer whose hand was always exposed to the sun as he drove about his work.

802 *The cautery* The hot cross on the skull given for severe headache and fevers in childhood.

800

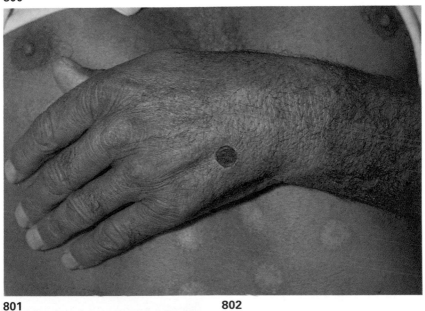

801

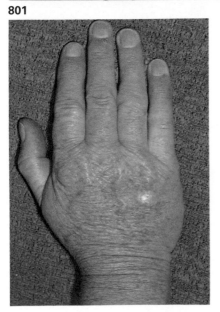

802

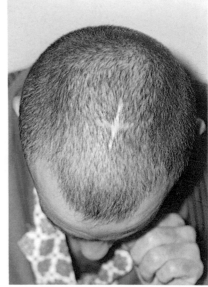

803 *Gallbladder pain* The cautery used for right sided upper recurrent abdominal pain – a case of gallstones.

804 *Chronic calculous cholecystitis (hot water bottle burn)* A similar end result with different beginnings in this woman who hugged a hot water bottle as a counter irritant for her gall bladder pain – she burnt herself!

805 *The cautery in the irritable bowel syndrome* Recurrent abdominal colic investigated in London and treated along conservative lines. The patient was unimpressed and on his return home underwent the cautery with remission of symptoms!

806 & 807 *The cautery in backache (L4/5 disc prolapse)* The scars from cautery are common as the pain is chronic and the sufferer will try anything in the hope of cure. Since his backache relapses and remits there is a good chance of the cautery getting the credit.

This 45-year-old policeman had low back pain (**807**) and had a combination of counter irritant cautery and therapeutic tattooing; there is no doubt about the site of the pain. On coughing and straining the pain radiated down the leg in an L5 segmental distribution (**806**). At the ankle there was impairment of sensation to pin prick which probably accounts for the severity of the cautery burn.

803

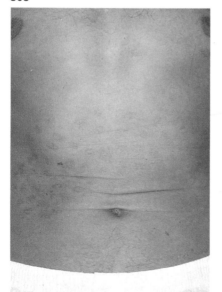

804

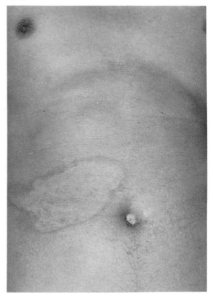

805

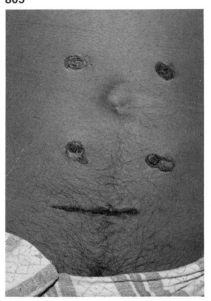

806

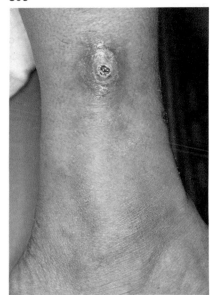

807

808 *The use of cautery in febrile convulsions* Sometimes in West Africa the child who has a febrile convulsion is thought to be the victim of an evil force in the body. The parent believes that immediate action to dislodge the evil and stop the twitching is necessary. The method is to plunge the feet into a cooking pot of oil. The twitching stops but leads to unpleasant burns of the feet. Feet such as these are pathognomonic of a convulsion which may be denied by the parent. It is not enough to treat the feet: the cause of the convulsion must be found and treated.

809 *Osteoarthritis* The site of the pain over the anterior attachment of the medial cartilage is given away by the scarification tattoo on the knees.

810 *Cupping* This is a common practice in Europe and the Near East though not seen in Africa. The round bruise marks on the back are caused by suction from round cups which are flamed inside with a taper and then applied to the back – as the cup cools it becomes firmly fixed to the skin and sucks blood to the surface. It can be combined with scarification before application of the cup – the suction then sucks blood into the cup. It is felt that the dark blood removed contains the toxins causing the illness, be it influenza, bronchitis or pneumonia. This therapy is most frequently used for acute febrile illnesses and the patient may present with an unresolved pneumonia and the marks.

808

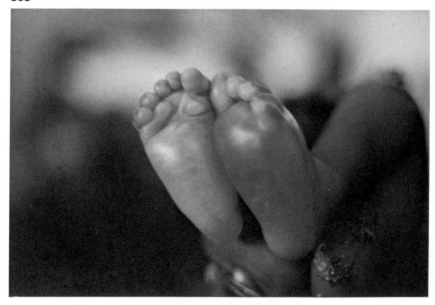

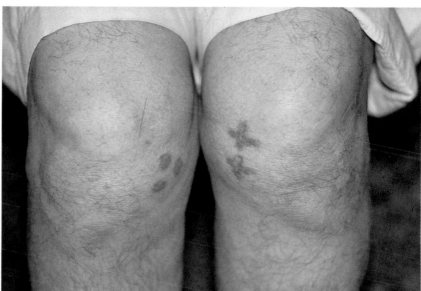

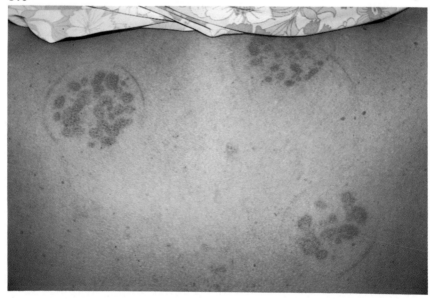

811 *Uvulectomy* Hausa surgeons in Northern Nigeria may remove the uvula for a variety of inflammatory conditions in the throat. It should not be confused with **812**.

812 *Scarred palate* Uvulectomy should not be confused with a scarred palate due to healed secondary syphilis or with a gumma.

811

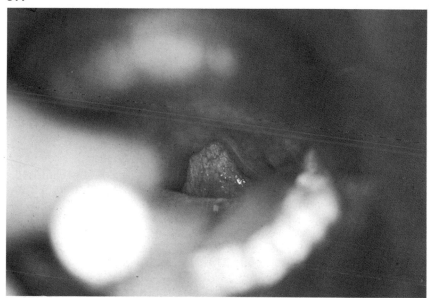

812

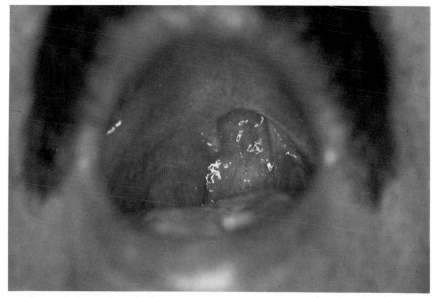

Acknowledgements

I thank my friends who have helped to fill in the gaps – I am indebted to them for the generosity in parting with slides. Dr Geraint James, my old chief, sparked my interest; Dr Anthony Dawson, Dr Alan Walker and Dr Kevin Zilkha spent many hours discussing what should be included and provided many superb slides. Dr Bill Clarke read the proofs, for which I am very grateful. I would also like to thank my two secretaries, Mrs Judy Stevens and Mrs Susan Chrimes, who typed and re-typed the manuscript and without whose help the book would not have been possible.

I am very grateful for the loan of the following illustrations: Sir Francis Avery Jones, **338**; Dr R Bayliss, **105–110**, **369**; Mr T R Bull, **162**, **313**, **317**, **327**, **373**, **374**, **383**, **539–541**, **545**, **546**; Dr C D Calnan, **700**, **706**, **767**, **775–778**; Dr L S Carstairs, **580–582**; Mr A Catterall, **288**, **534**; Dr R D Catterall, **347**, **366**; Dr W E Clarke, **342**, **343**, **629**; Dr A M Dawson, **339**, **340**, **542**, **642**, **643**, **662–664**, **669**, **670**, **674**, **675**; Dr M Dynski-Klein, **334**; Mr F G Ellis, **459**, **572**, **573**, **716**; Dr P Emerson, **707**; Dr R T D Emond, **754**; Dr P Evans, **63–65**; Dr C Harmer, **362**, **563**, **564**; Mr R Haskell, **204**, **363–365**; Dr D G James, **205**; Dr W M Jamieson, **378**; Dr H Jolly, **66**; Mr L W Kay, **204**, **363–365**; Dr G M Levene, **700**, **706**, **767**, **775–778**; Dr N McIntyre, **298–300**; Mr A Mushin, **309**, **310**; Dr I Sarkany, **191**, **196**, **212**, **213**, **223**, **224**; Dr M Spittle, **559–562**, **637**, **638**, **641**; Mr R Sweetnam, **286**, **287**, **693**; Dr A Walker, **68–70**, **240**, **241**, **496**, **523**, **574**, **618**, **683**, **718**; Wellcome Trustees, **732**; Dr A Wisdom, **348**; Dr I Zamiri, **387**; Dr K J Zilkha, **137**, **138**, **214**, **257–259**, **533**.

Index

(References printed in medium type are to page numbers and those in **bold** are to picture and caption numbers.)